the Orgasmic diet

the O

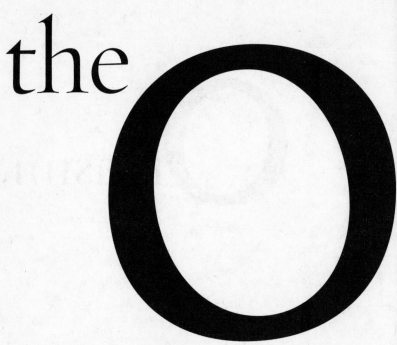

A Revolutionary Plan

to Lift Your Libido and

Bring You to Orgasm

 CROWN PUBLISHERS • NEW YORK

rgasmic
diet

MARRENA LINDBERG

TO STEPHEN COLBERT,
A TRUE FEMINIST, AND THE HOST OF THE
ONLY TELEVISION SHOW TO HAVE SHERE
HITE, GLORIA STEINEM, ARIEL LEVY,
LINDA HIRSHMAN, ARIANNA HUFFINGTON,
AND NORA EPHRON AS GUESTS.

Acknowledgments

I have a lot of people to thank for helping me, Dr. David Ferguson first of all. He took me seriously when everyone else thought I was crazy. He's freely helped me every step of the way, particularly in trying to get a study started. He's pushed me to dig deep and understand the science underlying my discovery. His generous, giving heart and rigorous mind have given me the encouragement to keep going on this quest of mine, to tell women.

And of course the second thanks must go to the women themselves. The positive support and encouragement I've received from the women (and men, too, but that story is for another book) who have tried the diet has been overwhelming. Hearing back from them about how I have changed lives, saved marriages, and brought pleasure has made all my work worthwhile. In some ways I'm the luckiest woman in the world—it's as if I'm living a secret *It's a Wonderful Life.* The whispered heartfelt thanks from women all over the world have given me the courage to get out there in public and talk, and keep talking, about what I've discovered.

I owe a particular thank-you to four women who early on wrote to me that they had already stumbled on a diet similar to mine with the same phenomenal sexual results—it really convinced me I was onto something.

I also want to thank the dozens of online message boards that have allowed me to spread the word about my plan to women worldwide, especially fsdinfo.org and bermansexualhealth.com. Also, the feedback from men's boards, in particular thundersplace.org, has been intensely encouraging. The men, the husbands and boyfriends of the women, sending their thanks has really cheered me.

And Tom Robbins's supportive response to my questions especially gave me courage and the certainty I was on the right path.

I also want to thank Oprah Winfrey for doing her show on vaginal cone weights, which was the last step in my accidental diet and triggered the startling results that made me sit up and take notice of the changes in my body. And I want to thank her staff for choosing my e-mail to be read on her show—that choice was the early encouragement I needed to keep going.

Dr. Irwin Goldstein and Dr. Andre Guay have my appreciation for giving me personal encouragement early on, and an education in the realities of medical research. And Dr. Joseph Hibbeln has been so tremendously supportive and reassuring, and a goad to keep me going when I've wanted to give up—I owe him so much.

I want to thank my family, particularly my daughters, for putting up with this time-consuming crusade of mine. I hope as they get older they will understand why I am making such a public spectacle of myself.

I owe a lot to the many people who have hotly debated with me. They have forced me to be rigorous and research the science showing I'm right and forced me to make my arguments more persuasive. In particular I want to thank the big pharma employee who told me I could never ever get a study going because I was a housewife. He gave me such a strong powerful anger, it really was a kick in the pants.

To Zoe Nelson at *Elle* magazine, who wrote such a wonderful and lengthy article about the Orgasmic Diet, searching me out and coming to my house and spending all morning talking, talking, talking—my personal fairy godmother—thank you. I hope you find what you are looking for.

I especially want to thank Carrie Thornton, my editor, who believed in this book from the very start and whose graceful guidance brought it to fruition.

Billie Fitzpatrick is my right arm—we wrote this book together, and I couldn't have done it without her. She balanced me in every area, with a sunny encouragement and warm assurance. I can't thank her enough. And I am grateful to Mary Ann Naples, for listening to me go on and on at the beginning, putting up with my naïveté, and for giving me a chance, showing me the ropes and what I needed to do. And of course, Debra Goldstein is the iconic ideal of agents, advising, opening doors, and confidently guiding me through this strange new world of publishing—thank you.

Inside I have changed, too, and those secret catalysts deserve open thanks. I want to thank the man who initially convinced me, really made me believe that there just might be men out there who truly like and respect very sexual women. If it weren't for that initial sea change, that saying yes to sex, I never would have been open to instinctively adopting my diet.

I really do hope that word about this program gets out to every woman because I think every woman deserves to know how her body works, sexually speaking. Every woman except for Tipper Gore—we can't be having Al Gore spending all day having tantric sex with his wife; he's got more important things to do right now. So shhhh!—don't tell her about this book. But everybody else—enjoy!

Medical Disclaimer

This book contains information about how to increase your ability to achieve an orgasm through a combination of diet, nutritional supplements, and exercise. While every care has been taken in researching and compiling the medical information in this book, it is not intended as a substitute for the advice and care of your physician, and you should use proper discretion, in consultation with your physician, in utilizing the information presented. The author and the publisher expressly disclaim responsibility for any adverse effects that may result from the use or application of the information contained in this book.

The Orgasmic Diet

"I would not give it up for money or threats!"

—Rita, 48, Washington

"I seem to be ready for sex now practically any time. I no longer need so much foreplay, and I initiate sex much more often."

—Paige, early 40s, California

"In two weeks, my libido increased. I was shocked by how low my libido had been before the diet!"

—Roberta, 36, Massachusetts

"Now, I am much more relaxed, less inhibited, and have a much easier time having an orgasm."

—Tracy, 30s, New York

"All orgasms are easier and yet more intense, and at times I have this ability to feel a clitoral orgasm to the very core!"

—Martina, mid-40s, Australia

"This is the diet for me—and my wife. I have never seen her so happy or ready for sex. The Orgasmic Diet has turned around our relationship!"

—John, mid-50s, Missouri

Contents

Contents

PART THREE

a truly satisfying sex life

Foreword

Women's sexuality is often described as "complex" in opposition to men's, and this is often the excuse for not correcting female sexual difficulties. The "it's-all-in-your-head" school of thought has prevailed all too long for women. In the case of men, the introduction of injection therapy and then oral drug therapy for erectile dysfunction (ED) made the it's-all-in-your-head concept ludicrous. The successes with men encouraged professionals working in the field of sexual medicine to anticipate the rapid introduction of pharmaceutical solutions to female sexual dysfunction (FSD). But that has not happened. Why? Factors contributing to female sexual dysfunction abound. Only recently, professionals have been teasing these factors apart, trying to assign relative degrees of importance. Common factors that appear to be prime culprits are stress, relationship issues, depression, disease, smoking, and drugs. The first three may be relieved by psychotherapy. But psychotherapy may not address physical issues. Medical practitioners, when willing to address FSD, are likely to prescribe medications. All too often, these drugs make the problems worse. What can be done?

Research on male sexual dysfunction revealed a number of interesting epidemiologic and pathologic connections. The commonly cited risk factors for heart disease were amazingly similar to those for ED. Subsequently, ED was identified as an early warning sign for heart disease. Erectile dysfunction also has been identified as a marker for what is called *cardiovascular metabolic syndrome:* the simultaneous presence of diabetes, hyperlipidemia, and hypertension. Atherosclerotic heart disease sometimes is included in that list also. What useful information can we derive from these discoveries?

The standard medical treatment for these conditions is diet and exercise, assuming that lifestyle choices are a major contributor to these diseases. If changes in lifestyle do not provide adequate correction of these conditions, then prescription drugs are added. Recently, epidemiology studies have strengthened the evidence that FSD may be connected to inappropriate diet and exercise and other lifestyle choices as well.

Diet and exercise. What does that mean? The subject of diet has long been plagued by fads, naysayers, conflicting data, and rampant misinformation.

Are there nutritional deficiencies or imbalances in modern countries today? It depends on whom you ask and whom you believe. In outpatient clinics, iron deficiency anemia and angular stomatitis (cracking of the corners of the mouth due to riboflavin, or vitamin B_2, deficiency) are seen routinely every day. Osteoporosis, partially due to calcium and vitamin D deficiency, is epidemic, especially among women. Prescription drugs like Fosomax have caused scurvy, or vitamin C deficiency. Type 2 diabetes mellitus (the non—insulin dependent kind) is becoming a major health and financial issue in the United States. Even children are getting it. Obesity, a risk factor for type 2 diabetes, has become a major target of federal health and education programs. Fad dieters and vegans frequently suffer nutritional deficiencies, some irreversible. So what should we eat?

Physicians commonly tell patients that they will get all the vitamins and minerals they need from their everyday diet. There are some big assumptions in that advice. First, it assumes that the patient is making food choices that provide a "balanced," nutritionally sound diet. Second, it assumes that the foods the patient chooses are complete, containing the full complement of vitamins and minerals necessary. Third, it assumes that the patient does not have a condition or take a medication that alters the nutritional requirements.

Let's address these assumptions. What is a balanced diet? The U.S. Department of Agriculture publishes "food pyramids" advocating that we consume certain quantities of different foods. It is interesting that these recommendations are from the same agency that oversees farm subsidies and agricultural surpluses. Similarly, the USDA advice changes frequently in response to less-than-definitive new scientific evidence. Most recently, the USDA couldn't settle on one food pyramid; it published twelve. How can the public "know" what to eat in this climate? The American Heart Association publishes "healthy" diets, yet it also endorses "Heart Healthy" foods such as Count Chocula. The apparent conflicts of interest exhibited by these organizations make their recommendations suspect. Low-fat diets heavy in grains have been advocated for decades, yet even patients who follow them have difficulty avoiding obesity, type 2 diabetes, and heart disease. Medical renegades like Robert Atkins analyzed these discrepancies and formulated seemingly paradoxical diets that purposely reduce carbohydrates (sugars and starches), promote proteins and vegetables, and suggest only moderate fat restrictions. Surprisingly, these diets work to reduce obesity, diabetes, and hyperlipidemia. As the role of insulin is further elucidated, the medical community is accepting these findings more and more.

Do people make healthy food choices, and do their choices contain all the nutritional factors they need? Studies show that fewer than 50 percent of households actually cook meals prepared from raw ingredients on a daily basis. Rather, they eat commercial "foods" like Hot Pockets, frozen pizza, carryout, and microwave dinners. Examination of the labels on these products clearly shows that they are high in fats and carbohydrates and low in protein. Current labeling requirements provide little information about vitamins and minerals. Large numbers of working people eat "fast foods" for lunch every day. Labels show these foods to be very high in fats and cereal-based carbohydrates. Even those who cook their own food from fresh ingredients face the issue of nutritional content. So much of our produce is grown on irrigated land that is only replenished with chemical fertilizer containing nitrogen, phosphate, and potash. Little or no attempt to replenish minerals and trace elements is made in large-scale farming. The result is flavorless, nutritionally deficient produce. Animals commercially raised for meat (including fish) are fed grain to boost their growth and weight for the best return on the dollar. The types of fat in these meats are not as healthy as those found in free-range animals.

Many conditions or medications can alter nutritional requirements. For example, menstruation can lead to loss of iron. Diabetes increases the need for calcium and potassium. Heavy exercise and the use of bottled water increase the need for calcium and magnesium. Pregnancy and nursing increase the need for folate and essential fatty acids. Antihistamines cause dehydration, thus increasing the need for minerals and water. Certain antibiotics can interfere with the absorption and/or utilization of vitamins. Stress increases the need for antioxidants.

Another factor that needs to be addressed is the metabolic and physiologic effects of different foods. The stimulant effects of coffee, tea, and chocolate have been known for centuries, but the exact mechanisms have only been recently understood. Among other things, these foods increase levels of dopamine in the brain, creating sensations of reward and pleasure. Other foods, such as carbohydrates, increase levels of serotonin in the brain. Some drugs (like antidepressants) can also raise serotonin levels. These drugs are associated with strong negative effects on sexual response. In fact, the serotonin-specific reuptake inhibitor class of antidepressants (SSRIs) is used to treat premature ejaculation. Certain fats also lead to stimulation of the brain, while others lead to satiety and sedation.

So what does all of the preceding have to do with sex? Simply put, your body can't function properly if it doesn't get the right nutrition. Deficiencies must be corrected. For sexual responsiveness, the body needs proteins and certain fats, but excess carbohydrates should be avoided. Minerals and trace elements can alter the body's response to drugs and underlying conditions.

Marrena Lindberg has developed a program of diet and exercise that alleviates the suppression of sexual response suffered by far too many women. She has carefully explored factors first on herself and then on other women who volunteered to try her methods. The results have been impressive! Currently, sexual experts encourage "evidence-based medicine." This means there should be solid evidence for assertions of treatment success. Typically, new advances in medicine start with observations followed by collection of case histories. Eventually, randomized, replicated, double-blinded, placebo-controlled studies are expected to "prove" the treatment. Ms. Lindberg has done the first step. I, and others, have tried to get her program into a well-controlled clinical trial, but so far we have been unable to find a sponsor to fund it. Since her program cannot be patented, there is little commercial interest in supporting such a study. One should keep in mind that many wonderful medical discoveries were made and accepted based solely on case histories; Banting and Best won the Nobel Prize for treating two diabetes patients successfully. Ms. Lindberg's results speak for themselves.

—David M. Ferguson, PhD, MD
Fellow, American College of Clinical Pharmacology
President, The Women's Sexual Health Foundation
Director at Large, International Society for the
Study of Women's Sexual Health

the Orgasmic diet

Introduction

If you're like me, with a busy life filled with raising kids, working hard at a job, and trying to keep your house clean, you probably struggle to find the time and energy for sex—whether you have a partner or not. And even when you do have time, you might, like millions of other women, have great difficulty feeling sexual desire, having an orgasm, or experiencing any sexual satisfaction at all.

You may think that all you need to fix this absence of passion and pleasure is time: time to get a massage, take a yoga class, be romanced by your sweetheart, or take a long bubble bath. That should do it, you believe, listening to the many voices out there who have you convinced that the key to embracing your sexuality is simply mind over matter. Well, nothing could be further from the truth.

I'm not saying female sexuality isn't complicated. We women like to be relaxed, aroused, and seduced—and sometimes all three. We have many different ways to experience sexual pleasure and can reach orgasm through various means. But the fact remains: if certain biochemical and physical pathways are not working exactly right, no amount of romancing we receive will ever get us to feel desire and achieve orgasm. Indeed a large percentage of women either cannot have an orgasm, have great trouble reaching orgasm, and/or experience little or no libido at all. These women are not unusual; they are actually suffering from female sexual dysfunction (FSD), which is defined as the inability to orgasm or difficulty in doing so, low or nonexistent libido, the loss of sensation and sexual responsiveness, and pain with intercourse. (Pain with intercourse is the only form of FSD not addressed by the Orgasmic Diet; if you are experiencing painful intercourse, it is advisable to see a medical professional.) And according to one recent study, 43 percent of women have some form of FSD; that's 50 million women in the United States—an astounding number!

The Orgasmic Diet will change all of that.

Not every woman who hasn't experienced an orgasm has FSD; some have just not been shown how to have an orgasm—clitoral or vaginal. Many women come to me saying, "I have never had an orgasm. I wouldn't know the difference between a vaginal and a clitoral orgasm—I don't even know what an orgasm feels like!" If you are in that boat, don't think you are all that unusual. Most women who can orgasm experience clitoral orgasm, from stimulation of their clitoris (either manually, orally, or using a vibrator). Some rare women are physically unable to have clitoral orgasms, but most are. It you have never had a clitoral orgasm, read chapter 9. If you are already having them but want more and/or want to achieve them more easily—go on my diet.

Many women claim they have never experienced a vaginal orgasm, and many women say that they rarely feel interested in sex. That's where the Orgasmic Diet comes in. One woman in her midthirties, who has been married for twelve years, said that the most remarkable thing she discovered being on the diet was how the diet affects the body. She commented, "I was amazed at how low my libido was before the diet."

A woman in her late thirties who had very low libido and sexual response (the two main types of FSD) found that after only two weeks following the diet, she had more interest in sex and pleasing her partner. She also said that the diet makes her feel "more relaxed, less inhibited," and that she had an easier time having orgasms. A woman in her early forties with two young children said, "Ever since the birth of my second daughter my libido has felt nonexistent. For the first year, it didn't really matter. But now my daughter is almost two and I am so frustrated. When I started taking the fish oil, I noticed a difference in almost three weeks! It was amazing— I was raring to go again! My partner was so relieved and grateful— he had his lover back again."

The Orgasmic Diet is a simple, straightforward nutrition and exercise program that will very quickly (in most cases women feel the effects in two weeks) have you willing, wanting, and able to have sex. In time you will be able to orgasm quickly and deeply—even during intercourse. Some women have been able to experience spontaneous orgasms, and others can climax within ten seconds of penetration. Essentially, the Orgasmic Diet can make you whatever kind of sexual dynamo you wish to be. This diet has not only worked for me and many other women who have tried it, so there is plenty of anecdotal evidence, but it is also backed up clearly by science.

One woman in her late forties recently told me that before going on the diet she was never able to reach orgasm during intercourse.

Within four weeks, she said she and her husband "went from ending nearly every sexual encounter in tears to acting like a couple of newlyweds." She added, "We have gone from going through the motions quickly three to four times a month to enjoying long, intense encounters three to four times each week! Our kids are coming home from college this week for the winter break and we're really not looking forward to the loss of privacy!" What a change, right? Another woman said that the Orgasmic Diet was so positive that she not only experienced "improved mood, libido, and lubrication" but also "more confidence and less inhibitions."

Nothing short of revolutionary, the Orgasmic Diet is the first-ever scientifically supported nutritional and exercise method to improve libido and orgasmic ability in women. So many books are written today about women and sex, and by far the greatest number deal with ways of getting in the mood or fixing relationships, or offer techniques for overcoming your inner boredom, reluctance, feelings of unattractiveness, or exasperation at how long it takes you to orgasm. And then there are many useful and informative books about technique—how to give yourself an orgasm, types of foreplay, special positions for sex, et cetera. All these books offer some helpful hints about reconnecting with your inner sexual self or your partner, but none fully addresses why your body is not able to have an orgasm or feel libido. *The Orgasmic Diet* addresses these problems. How do I know it works? Because I created the diet and have witnessed the life-altering effects it has had on me and hundreds of other people around the world. Just take another look at the testimonials that opened the book! And these women are offering just a taste of the powerful changes in sexual pleasure and desire you can experience with the Orgasmic Diet. This diet not only has the power to give women back their sexual health and ability to enjoy sexual pleasure, but it also has the potential to transform their lives, giving those who try it hope, confidence, and a renewed belief in themselves.

One of the features that makes my diet so different is that it enables you to learn how to have a vaginal orgasm. A vaginal orgasm feels different from a clitoral orgasm. First of all, women experience a vaginal orgasm within their vaginas. For some women, this sensation emanates from stimulation of the G-spot or cul-de-sac; other women experience a vaginal orgasm in a more general way when the entire muscle cavity begins to pulsate. Because my diet helps improve the connection between vulva and brain, helping women really *feel* the improved muscle strength, increased circulation, and enhanced tightness during sex, they become more able to have vaginal orgasms.

The Orgasmic Diet will improve both clitoral and vaginal orgasms, just in different ways. Clitoral and vaginal orgasms feel different because they emanate from different places. The clitoral orgasm is experienced very specifically in the clitoris; whereas the vaginal orgasm begins deep in the vagina, but spreads outward in feeling. Clitoral orgasms are sharper and more intense, vaginal orgasms are deeper and more full-body. One type of orgasm does not replace the other; in fact, the more of one kind a woman has, the more she may find herself wanting the other kind. They work together.

The Orgasmic Diet is all about increasing your ability to experience sexual pleasure. A woman who was forty-eight when she started the Orgasmic Diet found it changed her life. Married for twenty-five years and the mother of two children in college, she explained that she had become bereft when she began losing clitoral sensitivity. "Over time it became impossible for my husband to bring me to climax and difficult for me to get there on my own, even with a powerful vibrator. After some time on the Orgasmic Diet, I began to regain a little clitoral sensitivity, but the more remarkable thing was that I started having vaginal G-spot orgasms, including ejaculatory and spontaneous ones. This was entirely new for me."

If you've never had a vaginal orgasm, this diet will change that. If you are already having them, great, but now you'll have them faster and stronger. You can also learn how to increase the ease and intensity of your clitoral orgasm. You can now rev up your sex drive to match your partner's, even outdo him. Wouldn't it be nice to turn the tables and have your partner begging for a day off? Some women on the Orgasmic Diet have reported an extreme response: having a vaginal orgasm from only ten seconds of penetration, no foreplay required, and can keep on having them through the entire sex act. All of this—and more—may be within your reach, simply by following the four easy steps of the Orgasmic Diet.

The individual elements of the Orgasmic Diet are not medically controversial in any way. Each has already been proven to work individually, but the effectiveness of combining them had not yet been discovered—until I did. And although you can find all the scientific data that support the four individual steps of the diet in the Bibliography at the back of the book, no one yet—no scientist, no medical doctor, no sex counselor, no dietitian—has put these four elements together to not only address the main physiological roots of FSD but also renew passion and desire in women's lives.

Though the Orgasmic Diet is medically sound, part of the reason the Orgasmic Diet has not been shared sooner is because of the restricted point of view of many medical professionals. In general, FSD is treated by the medical community as a psychological problem, and women looking for help are referred to some sort of counselor, including marital counselors, sex counselors, and sometimes psychiatrists. Of course some of the causes for women's FSD can be psychological or relationship related, and therapy or counseling is appropriate. However, in my experience and research, many cases of dietary and nutritional women's FSD is physical in nature, and therefore women's bodies respond much more effectively to the elements of the Orgasmic Diet. Which is why when patients with FSD consult psychiatrists, they can just make matters worse: psychiatrists more than likely will treat a woman's depression with medications that simply exacerbate the problem.

Doctors are often less focused on nutritional ways to improve female sexual function; the fact is, most doctors are not trained in nutrition. They don't know that fish oil increases dopamine levels. They don't know that zinc and magnesium reduce sex-hormone-binding globulin. When I tell them and show them the studies proving these things, many get excited. The modern focus on pharmaceuticals often prevents the embracing of new, more holistic ideas about treating FSD and many other medical conditions. I have proof that my diet works from both animal and human studies and from the always growing amount of anecdotal evidence from women who have successfully tried it. It works in a healthy, holistic, and synergistic way, and in many ways re-creates the diet prehistoric humans ate. And, it simply makes sense.

Essentially, the Orgasmic Diet is based on four essential factors that influence and enable healthy sexual functioning in women:

1. Sufficient free testosterone

2. Balanced dopamine-serotonin levels

3. PC (pubococcygeus) muscle tone

4. Healthy genital circulation

The Orgasmic Diet improves all four of these aspects, enabling high sexual desire and intense sexual responsiveness in the process. Here's how the Orgasmic Diet works:

✳ It raises free testosterone through emphasis on high protein and increased levels of zinc and magnesium in your diet.

✳ It balances the levels of two important neurotransmitters regulating women's libido and sexual functioning, specifically dopamine and serotonin, through an increase of the omega-3 fatty acids found in fish oil supplements.

✳ It further boosts dopamine (the neurotransmitter enabling women to experience sexual pleasure) with healthy amounts of dark chocolate.

✳ It keeps serotonin from spiking and interfering with a proper serotonin-dopamine balance, by decreasing or altogether eliminating caffeine and all-carb meals.

✳ It improves blood flow to the genital region with the procirculatory benefits of fish oil, and it increases vaginal muscle tone through targeted exercise.

While a formal study of the diet has yet to be done (and I have begun the formal procedure for acquiring support for my research protocol), I *have* garnered medical and professional support from experts in the field. The director of a renowned FSD clinic at Columbia University signed on as a principal investigator for a study, and one of the foremost experts on fish oil at the National Institutes of Health (NIH) is also assisting me in my attempts to attract study funding. So know that this book's recommendation of fish oil as a supplement will be supported by the most up-to-date research available at the time of publication. Although I am not a medical doctor, I have been vigilant in having many in the medical community review the tenets of the Orgasmic Diet and have received unequivocal support. I have also found that the diet not only helps libido, but also improves general health for many; it is good for you.

High levels of dopamine do improve female libido, so much so that several dopamine drugs to treat female sexual dysfunction are currently in Phase I clinical trials. High levels of serotonin do decrease sexual function—antidepressants are already being prescribed for premature ejaculation, and the crippling antisexual side effects of anti-depressants for women are well documented, and an active field of research for the medical community. Free testosterone does control desire, and the number of women getting off-label (i.e., prescription drugs that are not yet approved by the FDA) testosterone replacement therapy (TRT) to help with FSD and the enormous popularity of books on the topic attest to how widespread and generally accepted it is, to the point where it has generated a backlash movement among some sex therapists at the blanket use of TRT for all women, no matter their case histories. Pubococcygeus (PC) muscle tone has already been proven to help female sexual response, especially with a high correlation to vaginal orgasmic ability. And finally, the importance of good genital blood circulation is now also widely accepted. There wasn't enough evidence for Viagra to pass clinical trials for women, but there is certainly enough anecdotal evidence of women out there "borrowing" their husbands' little blue pills and enjoying the results to make the idea that it would help women plausible.

The Orgasmic Diet is quite simple: eat a diet high in protein, low in carbs, and moderate in particular fats. Take fish oil supplements and some vitamins and minerals, reduce or eliminate caffeine consumption, eat a good amount of dark chocolate, and exercise your PC muscles. That's it. There is nothing outlandish about the diet; everything a woman needs can be purchased at her supermarket or local drugstore, except for the PC muscle exercise device, a $40 item easily purchased online. There is nothing exotic in my diet like yohimbe or bromocriptine, no strange herbs like Muira puama or valerian. In fact there are no herbs at all; the diet consists of common vitamins and minerals and foods many of us are already eating, or should be. The only rather unusual things in the Orgasmic Diet are the recommendations for eating dark chocolate and consuming lots of fish oil, but chocolate and fish have been eaten (and overeaten) and studied for centuries. And really, don't you want someone telling you to eat chocolate every day because it's good for you?

The Orgasmic Diet is very easy to live with, much easier to follow than a weight-loss diet, and the results are much more fun. And you can tailor the diet to your liking. One woman in her midthirties did not feel the need to use the PC exercise device because doing her Kegels was enough to strengthen her PC muscles for "sensational orgasms." Another woman doesn't like dark chocolate (!) so simply relied on diet changes and fish oil to experience a full range of orgasms. You can even adapt the diet to your needs, depending on how sexually intense you want to feel on any given day. (You'll find sample menus beginning on page 79.)

Even women who want to decrease their sex drive for various reasons can benefit from this knowledge; that is, if they want to tone down their libido and curtail their sexual responsiveness, then by all means, they can do the opposite of what the Orgasmic Diet recommends. But by and large, all the women who have tried the Orgasmic Diet have found that they enjoy feeling like very sexual beings, and they remain on the diet even between relationships. The fortysomething woman from New York who had never experienced a vaginal orgasm before trying the Orgasmic Diet said that she gained a new self-confidence from the diet: "Even walking down the street I noticed that I made eye contact with men more often and noticed a marked difference in their reaction to me. I even got propositioned on the subway three times in my second week on the diet!" And others have also found that being on the Orgasmic Diet leads to increased male interest in them, perhaps because men can sense the strong sexual interest that the Orgasmic Diet gives these women.

However, the women who will find the Orgasmic Diet an absolute godsend are the millions of women suffering from female sexual dysfunction (FSD). In short, women with low sexual functioning will find the Orgasmic Diet an answer to their prayers, and women who already have *good* sexual function will find the Orgasmic Diet brings them *great* sexual function. Women are tired of hearing "Take a bubble bath." They want a straightforward solution to their sexual problems with obvious results, and that solution is the Orgasmic Diet.

the science of sex

PART ONE

CHAPTER ONE

How I Created the Orgasmic Diet

Why am I writing this book? There's one simple reason: because my diet will make you feel like a goddess—a sex goddess. And you should know about it because it has the power to change your life. As I stated in the introduction, the diet works, works well, and works quickly. It will give you back your sexual power and enable you to feel sensual pleasure, orgasms, and the ripple of desire— when and how you wish.

But before I give you all the information you will need to access the sexual goddess within you, I want to share a bit about myself and how this diet came to be. I want to share this story not to broadcast the ups and downs of my life, but because I think that many women can relate to my experience, specifically to my (former) great difficulty having orgasms and feeling sexual pleasure, and how that one thing missing in my life led me first to the depths of low self-esteem, bad choices, and chronic depression and then to a life full of joy, confidence, and boundless pleasure and fun.

From the Outside Looking In

Nine years ago I had it all—or at least I had convinced myself that I had it all. I was married to a man to whom I was devoted. We both had good jobs; we were doing extremely well in the stock market and looking to buy a house as soon as he finished his PhD in theology. He was the perfect man. He was romantic, thoughtful, prone to spontaneously buying me flowers, fun, smart, witty, in terrific shape, and very good-looking. Our home was filled with antiques and beautiful oriental rugs, thanks to his side job dealing in them, and he was doing important and seminal work for our church. I was very proud of him. I loved him body and soul. We were planning on having a baby.

But the sad truth was, I was miserable, and for a long time, I didn't really know that about myself. I didn't know that I had lost my center, given up my power, and given all of me away. You may be wondering why, if my life looked so good from the outside, I was so miserable. The answer lies in my sexuality.

In my marriage there was a fundamental inequality of power, an inequality hidden behind bedroom doors. I had always had trouble reaching a clitoral orgasm, but this inadequacy soon grew into a source not only of marital strife but also of seething insecurity for me. Soon after we were married, my husband began to tire of the extreme difficulty he faced in bringing me to orgasm; it took me a very long time. He would sigh and roll his eyes, which, of course, completely killed it for me. After the first year, I stopped asking him to pleasure me, and even when he occasionally asked if I wanted to have an orgasm, I was so ashamed I just snapped back no. Soon foreplay dwindled because it became easier to endure sex if I didn't get aroused. Getting aroused and not having an orgasm was worse than just lying there and feeling nothing.

There came a point when it had been more than five years since my husband had given me an orgasm, and more than six months since I had given myself one. I was sexually shutting down. Yet in a desperate attempt to keep my husband sexually satisfied, I would consent to sex—despite my having no desire or feeling whatsoever. Our infrequent interludes began to feel like invasions, degrading to both of us. Here was a man who was better than most at the skills of foreplay and who delighted in the erotic, now reduced to little more than a robot. And here I was, crumbling in shame at my own inadequacies and shortcomings, going through the motions, and unable to speak up on my own behalf.

Opening My Heart to Questions of Desire

And then something in me began to change. I asked myself, "Is your heart open to sexual pleasure? Is your heart open to change? Are you willing to kindle something inside that might be hard to hold on to?" Some part of me was gasping for life, for a chance to breathe. I began to realize that I had to be willing to believe that I was capable of both feeling sexual and having an orgasm. But I needed a partner. And since my husband and I had become so estranged in the bedroom, I created an imaginary man, a phantom, a Greek god. I needed an imaginary man who was infinitely patient, skilled at foreplay, relaxed, nonjudgmental, and completely focused on female pleasure for its own sake, but also contrarily not focused at all; a sort of dreamy diffusion of a man who kept his pants on, his eyes open, and his mind languorous. This man wanted nothing more than to please me and I didn't have to worry about pleasing him. I kept the idea of this man in my mind's eye, and the sexual frost that had lasted so long within me started to thaw.

I still felt like a sexual cripple, but in my imagination I had a man who was turned on by me exactly as I was. I was still sleeping with my husband (we wanted to have a baby), and instinctively I began making pro-sexual choices. Unwittingly I started out on my path of discovering the Orgasmic Diet.

I wanted to get pregnant, but I was on antidepressants, so I researched natural ways of treating depression and learned how vitamins, minerals, and foods influenced neurochemistry, particularly how protein, fats, and carbohydrates interacted with one another and the brain. As a result, I changed my diet. I then weaned myself off antidepressants under my doctor's supervision. With diet and exercise I managed to hold my depression at bay without the help of drugs. Getting off antidepressants alone was a huge help for my libido, of course, but the changes in my diet started having an effect, too. My libido not only picked up, it took off. Unbeknownst to me, I was creating a program. I still wasn't having orgasms, but at least during sex I was feeling something. Gone was the sensation of being an unmoving and unmoved receptacle. I was thrilled, and my husband was, too.

I got pregnant and was soon about to discover the three other elements of my diet. Of course, I quit drinking coffee and avoided all other stimulants. I also grilled my natal nutritionist on the most current research about fetal brain health. I was worried my baby might inherit depressive tendencies that were apparent on both sides of the family. My nutritionist strongly recommended fish oil,* and I started taking a megadose within the first couple months of my pregnancy.

---

* As every woman is different, you should consult with your gynecologist/obstetrician before taking fish oil during pregnancy or nursing. If you do decide to take fish oil, make sure to only get the highest quality, ultra-refined fish oil (see chapter 4 for further information).

It's not unusual for some women to experience an increase in libido during pregnancy due to hormones, so at the time, I chalked up my jump in libido and sexual ability to my pregnancy and didn't think much of it. After my first child was born and I was breast-feeding, I saw my libido drop just like most every breast-feeding mother's does—lactation hormones are Mother Nature's birth control. But I knew something was up when my libido came roaring back after I weaned her.

When I got pregnant with, breast-fed, and then weaned my second child, I watched my body go through the same cycle of high libido and active sexual response during pregnancy to a dip while I was nursing, and then a dramatic roar-back once I had weaned. Both through the pregnancies and after, I continued with the high-dose fish oil, vitamins, minerals, and a 40 percent carbs-30 percent protein-30 percent fat diet. I stayed off the coffee, and started eating dark chocolate, which I have always enjoyed. I had really begun enjoying the sex my husband and I were having—I wasn't about to give up now!

The final piece to the puzzle for me appeared after watching an episode of *The Oprah Winfrey Show* on vaginal cone weights. After two ten-pound babies, I knew I needed to get my muscle tone back; everything was stretched out down there. So following Oprah's advice, I began exercising with the vaginal cone weights. I was dedicated, working out at least twice a week, and soon I mastered the highest level.

And then something happened that completely blew me away. Driving home late one night after dropping off my girls at their grandmother's for an overnight, I had a long monotonous stretch of highway driving. Listening to the radio, I began to fantasize and reflexively flex my PC muscles. Twenty minutes of intricate fantasy later, and much to my shock, I had an orgasm. It was a different sort of orgasm than the clitoral kind, which had always required so much effort, further up and in. But what was this? How could I, a woman who needed such intense and prolonged stimulation to have an orgasm, all of a sudden have an orgasm with no touch whatsoever? You could have knocked me down with a feather. My first thought was, *My marriage is saved!* My second thought was, *I knew I was onto something.*

Yes, I was now enjoying sex and was enthusiastic because, on the diet, I began experiencing better sensation. But our marriage was suffering because I still could not have an orgasm during intercourse. I couldn't get away from that fact, and it rankled me at my very core. So we were still having brief sex with no foreplay, and I was still too insecure to ask for foreplay for fear that it would only lead to frustration, impatience, and feelings of inadequacy. But now this—this newfound ability to orgasm deep in my core was amazing—so why couldn't I put it all together? If I could hone this ability, surely I could have an orgasm from vaginal stimulation—I could have an orgasm just from sex!

I became a maniac. I started researching different ways to tone my PC muscles and became a weight-training fanatic—vagina-wise. I kept tinkering around with my diet, because after careful observation I noticed the orgasmic ability came and went depending on what I was eating, whether I took my fish oil or if I drank too much coffee. I became a sexual mad scientist, using myself as a guinea pig; I isolated the elements of my diet that were contributing to this magical vaginal orgasm ability, and I worked them.

With my mathematics training and my job at a science-focused environmental engineering firm, I approached my body and its responses as a scientist on a mission. I started doing research, investigating why these particular elements worked so well to produce such a magical effect. One by one I stopped and started, increased and decreased specific elements. And to my complete satisfaction, my experimentation bore fruit. Soon, instead of twenty minutes of intense fantasy, driving in a vibrating car, I was able to reduce it to fifteen, then ten, then five minutes simply from flexing and thinking, just sitting in a chair—and then, bang, I started orgasming during sex. I started having an orgasm with no foreplay, just from five minutes or less of receiving hard thrusting (and concentrating pretty hard). Suddenly orgasms were easy for me, a simple by-product of intercourse itself.

My husband was ecstatic! He felt incredibly studly! I was also ecstatic. And driven. After so many years of basically sexual voyeurism, even in the midst of sex, I was now a full and equal participant. I kept researching and tweaking and tinkering with myself. I developed my vaginal muscles even more, to a higher strength and greater coordination. I pushed my diet until my libido was in the stratosphere. Not only did I develop the ability to have dozens of spontaneous orgasms a day, I developed the desire to do so. Having an orgasm became as easy as breathing.

Just as I was beginning to relax into this pleasure, my husband began saying that he thought I had gone too far. He became very uncomfortable with the idea that he wasn't the one in control of giving me an orgasm. He was bothered by my being able to orgasm practically at will. He didn't enjoy it when I would have an orgasm from giving him oral sex. And he didn't like that I had an orgasm simply from him entering me.

And then our sex, which was infrequent at best, dwindled even further, and *he* started avoiding intercourse. Our rate of vaginal intercourse kept dropping, and for me, now having a very high libido, this was hard to bear. As long as I had thought that the fault was mine and believed that my body just didn't work like other women's, I could take the denial of pleasure, the starvation of touch. I used to accept this former lack of pleasure as the best I could expect. But now everything was different. Now I felt like a goddess. I felt inside that these newfound powers were perfectly wonderful and a cause for celebration—if only my husband could see it that way. But it was too late—our marriage dynamic could not change. I was still the dysfunctional one, the one with the problem. And I started seeing how this attitude had seeped out of the bedroom and into every aspect of our daily lives. I was wrong: we were not in an equal relationship and never would be, and I was not being treated well. I asked him to move out, and three years later we divorced.

The Silver Lining

But as with many bad experiences in our lives, this one had a hidden silver lining. After all of my experimentation and research, I realized I was truly onto something. Not something that was particular to me, to my body alone, but something that I knew would benefit other women, too. I already knew FSD was a big issue from talking with friends and of course from magazines, books, and movies. I knew this as well from dialoguing with hundreds over the Internet on message boards for women with sexual questions and issues; clearly, I was one of thousands—probably millions—of women who were unable to have orgasms and who struggled with low libido. If the diet could help me, it could also help others, so I searched online for communities of women getting together to discuss sexual difficulties and solutions, and I began posting at many such websites. I encouraged women to try my diet, and many did, having similar results. Some just had an increase in libido. Some developed vaginal orgasmic ability for the first time. Some learned to feel a clitoral orgasm more intensely. And some took it all the way and got to where I was. I was amazed.

These women became not only a source of support and encouragement, they became my inspiration. Seeing their heartfelt thanks and appreciation in e-mails from around the world made me feel that I was part of something larger, a community of women who wanted to feel sexual again, who wanted to feel empowered by their sexuality, and who were not going to settle for anything but a complete transformation in their physiology.

These anecdotal success stories meant the world to me, but I still wanted to get scientific support and approval for my diet. I naively thought if I could just tell sexuality researchers about my discoveries that they would jump at the chance to study it. I thought I had discovered the female Viagra. But although I got warm encouragement from the medical community, no one was willing to investigate an unproven approach for free. This galvanized me and I realized the only way research would be done on my diet was if I pushed it every step of the way. I thought if I popularized the diet it would be easier to get grant money. I pushed the diet very hard online and started investigating the possibility of writing a book. I researched the top doctors in the field, the grant foundations, good clinical trial practices, statistical analysis techniques. I started attracting attention and help from some of the top researchers in the field of sexual health. I explained the science behind each step of my diet and was able to persuade doctors of the validity of my approach. In many places I was challenged, and this was good for me. In defending my science I was forced to be completely rigorous and come up with references from studies and other supporting evidence.

Having an Ivy League math degree and having spent ten years working at a science and research—oriented environmental consulting company, I was in my element. As more and more women tried the diet, they enthusiastically gave me feedback, encouraging me to keep trying to get the word out. Even more encouraging, four women wrote to me saying they had discovered a very similar diet independently, with similar results. I knew I was right.

So to reiterate why am I writing this book—I am writing this book for you. In the movie *Kinsey* there was a woman like me, with my sexual abilities. She was a cheerful gray-haired grandmother. I am an equally improbable example of someone with advanced sexual skills—a plump suburban mom who wears sensible shoes. I've landed on my feet after my divorce. I have a good-paying programming job doing data mining—that math degree paid off after all. And I have found the key to my sexual bliss.

There is no earthly reason I should make a public spectacle of myself as "Spontaneous Orgasm Woman," except for the very important fact that I know something you need to know. I now know how women's bodies work, and I want you to know, too. You don't have to take the Orgasmic Diet to the extreme level I have; you can tailor it to fit your life, your relationship, and your sex drive. And while this knowledge may have blown up my own marriage, I firmly believe that it can save many others. I have already seen marriages healed from women putting my diet into practice. Also, I strongly hope that young women, who perhaps feel physically inadequate in the bedroom, like I used to, might come to realize both how normal they are and also how they can change this view of themselves and, if they desire, make sex easier and less stressful. Indeed, a woman who has a strong sexual response feels more powerful in her life and can make more empowering choices. I want to save women from feeling trapped the way I felt in my marriage, and I want to inspire them to reach for as much sexual power as they want.

Most important, I want all women everywhere to feel the pleasure and confidence that come from having healthy and balanced brain chemistry and good levels of hormones. My diet helps with that, and it has brought me inner joy, pleasure, and strength that I didn't know were even possible. I would like you to try it and see for yourself.

CHAPTER TWO

What the Orgasmic Diet Can Do for You

I strongly believe one fundamental truth—every woman is differ-ent. Every woman is different *especially* when it comes to sex. While the Orgasmic Diet helps sexual physiology, sex is more than just physiology. And even looking at the body's sexual response, every woman's body is unique.

I can give you a map to show you the lay of the land, how your body works, but only you can decide what path you will take. Women have very different sexual problems. Some women have never had a clitoral orgasm. Some women never feel the desire for sex, but once they are engaged in sex can easily have clitoral orgasms. Some women are too tense to be able to relax and enjoy sex. Some women feel that sex is bad and wrong and icky. Some women have very high libido and great clitoral orgasmic ability, but feel like there is something sexually wrong with them because the physical act of intercourse does nothing for them physically—inside the vagina they have about as much erotic sensation as they do on their elbows. Some women feel unloved. Some women feel unvalued. Some women are self-conscious about their bodies and feel unattractive. Some women deep down just don't find their partners sexually attractive anymore. Some women are breast-feeding and their lactation hormones have killed their sex drive. Some women have had their ovaries removed during a hysterectomy and have lost more than half of their testosterone-producing ability, like a man being castrated. Some women are mothers and feel it is unseemly for mothers to have a sex drive. Some women are on such an extreme vegan, nonfat, high-soy diet that their bodies, thinking it is a time of famine, have shut down their sexuality. Some women just naturally have low testosterone and have never understood all the hoopla about sex. Some women have lost all capacity for sensual pleasure. Some women have gone through menopause and their sex hormones have plummeted. And some women have secret desires that are not being satisfied.

What Happened to Me on the Diet

"In the past I had problems with vaginal dryness. On the diet, this has noticeably improved. My orgasms feel deeper, and my refractory period between orgasms has gotten shorter. My libido has always been tied to my hormonal cycle. I'm much hornier around the time I'm ovulating, while I'm not really interested in sex right before my period. This has not changed, but the horny period starts earlier and last much longer."

—Christa

Where You Fit In

How does my diet fit in with these myriad situations? How can I say one approach is best for all women? I can't, and I'm not going to. The irony is that the woman my diet will help the most is the woman least likely to be reading this book. Women who have never had libido can't figure out why on earth sex is so important to people. They want relationships, they want love, and they assume sex is just the price they have to pay. Curiously, women who have had strong libido in the past can lose their libido and feel exactly like this. It's a peculiar thing; I call it sexual amnesia, and I had it myself, many years ago before I went on my diet. You just forget the point of sex, the lure of sex. Sex becomes a chore.

However, the majority of women reading this book will be thinking more along the lines of "Why do my clitoral orgasms take so long to achieve?" or "Where has my libido gone?" or "Can I really have a vaginal orgasm just from intercourse?" My diet can help with all of those things—think of it as a sexual tune-up. So many women are where I was, loving the intimacy of having a man inside her, but wishing it felt a little more, well, anything. And even for the woman who is at her sexual peak, there's still further to climb if you're game. You can develop your vaginal muscles to have the tightness of a virgin's and the strong coordination to milk a man to orgasm, or develop your tantric kundalini energy to enable you to have chakra orgasms, or simply raise your libido to such a height that you both desire and are able to reach a tremendously multiorgasmic state.

You can use my diet in whatever way is best for you. Knowing the science of how your body works sexually may be enough, and you may choose to stay where you are or even dampen your sexuality by doing the reverse of my diet. Knowledge is power, and a woman who knows how her body works has power over her own sexuality. And I believe that sexual power, however she chooses to exercise it, is every woman's birthright.

Once women get the physical (biochemical) sexuality functioning in top form, something my diet is specifically aimed at doing, many of them just might also feel more empowered to get to the bottom of the subtle and complicated issues that inhibit a full expression of their sexuality.

In general my diet is helpful for most sexual problems that women have—not because it solves all sexual problems, but because it increases libido and makes it easier to have orgasms. When your desire is reawakened and you're able to experience the pleasure of an orgasm more easily, then you will feel more

What Happened to Me on the Diet

"I was forty-eight when I started (I am now fifty). I have always had a high libido and enjoyed sex a lot. I only ever climaxed through clitoral stimulation and never during intercourse, but it never bothered me. My husband always made sure I was satisfied before we had intercourse. I enjoyed intercourse, but not orgasmically. Over the previous couple of years, though, I discovered that I was gradually losing clitoral sensitivity. I believe it was related to perimenopause. After some time on the Orgasmic Diet, I began to regain a little clitoral sensitivity, but the more remarkable thing was that I started having vaginal/G-spot orgasms, including ejaculatory and spontaneous ones. This was entirely new for me. I can tell in the morning if I forgot to take the fish oil the night before—I miss my usual morning libido surge!"

—Tracy

motivated to solve the emotional or psychological issues that may be curtailing your sexual experience or lurking behind your relationship.

Honing in on Your Sexual Self

Despite my emphasis thus far on the body and physical approaches to fixing libido, I do strongly believe in the mind-body connection for women. Only you know deep down what your true sexual situation is. Women have an instinct about their bodies and their sexuality, and they should listen to that instinct. Only you know if your life makes you so stressed out that you have to live on a diet of Red Bull and coffee to keep up. Only you know if deep down you have given up on sex and are subconsciously desexualizing yourself with a constant diet of doughnuts and pasta. Or desexualizing yourself with a diet of tofu, soy milk, and rice cakes. Only you know deep down what truly turns you on, and what your deepest desires are.

Indeed, all women need to zero in on themselves, listen deeply to their inner voice, and learn to take care of themselves, and we need to do this regularly. What do you really need? Even after seven years on my diet, I still take care of myself in this way. Every month or so, I practice a relaxation exercise.

And as much as I have criticized the "bubble bath approach" to addressing women's sexual problems, I do rely on my own personal bath ritual as a way to get back in touch with myself and realign my sexual compass. I use this ritual as a way to create time for myself and to tune in to my inner sexual self.

The key thing about this exercise is that it causes a state of deep relaxation and very high dopamine levels; how you react to being in such a state, or if you can get there, will say a lot about your sexual response and ability to experience pleasure. So take a look at the

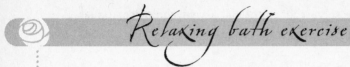

First off, you need time to yourself. That means kids and husband out of the house for at least three hours. I know, I know, nearly impossible, you say. But I'm not saying to do this all the time, maybe just once every month or two, to connect with your sexual subconscious and your body. Do whatever feels most comfortable and most relaxing. The important thing is to relax and let your mind wander, guiding it to wander in a sexual direction.

1. Turn up the heat. You want a toasty warm house.

2. Brew a pot of damiana tea. Women who are pregnant, nursing, or trying to get pregnant should not take damiana. If you are on any medications, check with your doctor before taking it. Damiana leaves are harvested from the plant *Turnera diffusa,* a small shrub native to Mexico, the American Southwest, and the West Indies. It has traditionally been used as a female aphrodisiac. You can find bulk damiana very cheaply online. Herbalist websites carry it; you should be able to get a few ounces for under five dollars. It is very easy to use a teaball and make tea from it. The taste is rather bitter; feel free to sweeten the tea with honey. If you feel uncomfortable with such a do-it-yourself approach, you can also buy damiana in capsule form at most drugstores. Just make sure to get pure damiana, not damiana mixed with some other herb like ginseng. Don't take damiana on a regular basis, and don't take it before driving or at any time you wouldn't want to be very relaxed and uninhibited.

3. Relax, put your feet up, drink the tea (or take a capsule or two), and read erotica for half an hour. There are lots of free and excellent erotica websites geared toward women. Professional websites like the Erotica Readers and Writers Association and Clean Sheets are excellent, and there is also a huge variety of amateur erotica online written by women, some at literotica.com and lots at fan fiction websites. Of course there is also wonderful erotica in book form. Read what you like, even if it's simply the steamy parts of a romance novel bought at your local supermarket. Whatever catches your imagination. (See the Resources section for details.)

4. Light a candle and take a bath. I recommend a scented candle and a scented bath. For the candle I recommend a vanilla-, rose-, or ylang-ylang-scented candle. For the bath my favorite add-in is the Body Shop's Ylang Ylang Bath Essence; very sensual. But whatever product you pick, don't pick something that is supposed to be soothing and sleep inducing or refreshing and citrusy. Pick a bath oil or bath salts that are packaged in red, that contain musk, patchouli, ylang-ylang, or sandalwood scents—something that is deliberately trying to be erotic.

5. After your hot bath, towel off, blow out the candle, and get into bed naked. Put on a sleep mask so that everything is dark and put on headphones. I strongly recommend listening to a Brainsync CD; I especially recommend the one titled *Ecstasy*. The Brainsync CDs are a line of music with a particular thrumming bass rhythm. The frequency of this rhythm, when listened to with headphones, tricks the brain into thinking it is hearing very deep sound waves below the human hearing range. This triggers changes in brain wave activity, leading to relaxed states similar to trance or hypnotic states, and also deep relaxation conducive to sleep. Some of the CDs have hypnosis or subliminal suggestion. The *Ecstasy* CD simply has music. You can order Brainsync CDs at www.brainsync.com.

description of the exercise and see how it works; it may be just what you need to open yourself to where you are sexually and what you need now, next month, or in your next relationship.

Basically I am recommending that you enter an altered state—but not a state of complete hypnosis like in the movies. Simply shut down your higher consciousness, your vision, and your hearing, so that all that is left is taste, touch, and smell. Wake up the senses you don't generally use—your sexual senses. Feel your body, the feel of the sheets on your naked body. Smell enticing smells. Deeply relax your mind and let your consciousness drift. And there, in that state, ask your subconscious about sex. What do you like? What do you want? What are you missing? Fantasize. If this process alarms you, ask yourself why. Explore your heart, explore your desires.

You aren't writing down these thoughts, you aren't telling a soul about your desires. You can think what you like in complete freedom, even if it's something completely taboo, like being dominated, or embarrassingly juvenile, like being rescued by a knight in shining armor. It doesn't matter whether your thoughts are silly or dirty or wrong or perverse or focused on someone besides your husband— they're secret, they're private, and they're just fantasy. Learn what makes you tick and listen to what your subconscious is telling you about your sexual state. Remember the path you took to your deepest desires, and it will be easier to get there again, even when you aren't relaxed or alone or drifting on damiana.

After all that, if you want to have an orgasm (or two), feel free, with toys or hands. Or call up your husband and tell him to come home right this instant! This isn't a sensate focus technique or a sexual technique really—it's just a way to awaken your body and your sexual mind.

Now let me ask you some questions:

* Did you immediately fall asleep as soon as you got into bed? Or did you spend the entire time worrying about your to-do list for tomorrow? My diet will help you, but you are also going to need to destress your life, get more relaxation time and more sleep. Perhaps your partner can help you if he is pressuring you for more sex.

* Did you have an orgasm even though in day-to-day life you never think of sex? My diet will definitely help you. It helps bring feelings of relaxation and pleasure into daily life. Instead of waiting for your partner to initiate sex before your body wakes up and you feel sexual pleasure, you will feel a blossoming of sensuality from the increased dopamine from the diet.

* Did you feel relaxed and sensual but not the slightest bit turned on? My diet may help you, but if it doesn't wake up your libido,

you may want to consider having your hormone levels tested, particularly your total and free testosterone.

❋ Did you feel really turned on and compelled to have an orgasm but couldn't? My diet will help you. It will help increase clitoral sensitivity, the ability to have vaginal orgasms, and libido in general. (Chapter 9, "Clitoral Orgasms 101," will help in particular with clitoral orgasms.)

❋ Did you feel panicked and upset? In this case, my diet may not help you. If your body and mind froze up at the thought of total relaxation and sexual fantasy, you may want to think about seeing a sexologist. (See the Resources section for more info on sexologists and counseling in general.)

❋ And finally, because I know there are women reading this book who already have great sexual function but want to take it as far as they can: Do you now want to throw me a ticker-tape parade after getting really turned on, having multiple orgasms, and then having a deep and refreshing nap? Well, go right ahead. And if you have great sex tips you'd like to share in return, post in my forum (www.orgasmicdiet.com). I always like to learn about new things! And go on my diet, because it will help you get your body into peak sexual form.

Recording Your Thoughts

Looking at how you (both your mind and your body) reacted to my relaxation technique can give you clues about the best way to approach my diet. The point is to begin to consciously cultivate and remember what turns you on. If you want to really know yourself sexually, it's a great exercise to actually write down your thoughts, feelings, and experiences—as they relate to sex. I've prepared a

What Happened to Me on the Diet

"I'm thirty-six and have been with my husband for fifteen years. Our sex life has always been pretty good, but I was always dependent on a vibrator for a clitoral orgasm. Then things between us started to go downhill. Because of a car accident, I began experiencing chronic pain and really lost my libido as a result. When I went on the Internet in search of information on the supposed "postthirties peak," I found the Orgasmic Diet and tried it. After two months on the diet, I have more sensitivity overall and a shorter time between orgasms, and my libido is greater. And, best of all, I'm no longer dependent on my vibrator for orgasm. Sex is just a much richer experience."

—Carey

Fantasy Worksheet for you to work from. You can also use a blank journal. Whatever works for you. Again, this exercise is about making a special effort to record your thoughts, fantasies, desires, and even your fears following the suggested relaxation exercise or whenever you want. In chapter 9, "Clitoral Orgasms 101," you can find specific suggestions for other ways to increase your erotic imagination and get more accustomed to unleashing your fantasies. But for now, approach this worksheet as a further way to get in touch with your sexual self.

Worksheet

Describe the most erotic dream you've ever had.

If you could have sex with anyone you choose, what would the perfect sexual partner look like, sound like, feel like—be like?

What would the sex with this ideal partner include?

What is the naughtiest thing you can imagine doing and enjoying sexually?

Describe the most erotic scent you can imagine.

What sort of touch gives you the most pleasure?

There are no right or wrong answers to the questions. You don't have to share the information with anyone. The Orgasmic Diet can work for you in many ways—it can definitely lead you to vaginal orgasms, increased libido, and more intense sexual responses; it will more than likely increase your pleasure in clitoral orgasms. But probably most important, the Orgasmic Diet is going to empower you with knowledge of yourself, in particular your sexual self. So now, before you dive right in and begin the diet, take some time to see that sexual self for who she is and what she wants.

CHAPTER THREE

How the Orgasmic Diet Works

As you have probably guessed by now, I am obsessed with science and research! This is one of the many reasons I feel so passionately about sharing the Orgasmic Diet—it not only works and works quickly, but it is also completely supported by science and current research.

I promise I won't bore you with long, dull scientific explanations about how the Orgasmic Diet works, but I do think you might be interested in getting a quick glimpse of how the diet actually impacts your body and brain and why it produces its marvelous results.

So if you'll put on your thinking cap for now, you'll enjoy that "nightcap" more later!

Dopamine: The Pleasure Transmitter

Imagine yourself on vacation. No kids, no job, no worries. You're a little bored, even. Lazing on a tropical beach, nothing much to do, you spend your day in pleasure. You eat superb food in restaurants and someone else does the dishes. And best of all, you are with a man and you are crazy in love with him. Just holding his hand makes your heart beat faster, and now you are spending all day with him, watching his muscular body diving into the surf, watching him towel himself off next to you. Later, you have a fabulous romantic candlelit dinner near the beach, with a glass of good wine, then you walk along the moonlit beach holding hands, and he takes you back to the hotel, lights a couple of scented candles, and gives you an expert rubdown over your entire body with warm sandalwood massage oil.

You've rolled over in perfect relaxed bliss, and you see him standing there, and he's ready, looking at you. How do you feel right at that minute? Do you want sex? That's dopamine at work, making you feel hot, horny, and ready.

Dopamine is one of many neurotransmitters that act as the brain's messengers, and it has a lot of jobs. It's a precursor to other neurotransmitters and also works as a hormone, suppressing prolactin, but its most important job is as the neurotransmitter of reward. Dopamine is the body's signal to itself that whatever activity was just done is a good one. It lights up the pleasure system of the brain and makes us feel good. Important evolutionary things like eating and sex are rewarded with dopamine release in the brain. It is also tied together with feelings of anticipation and desire. And, most important for us here and now, dopamine is one of the keys to libido because it is partly responsible for determining a woman's capacity for pleasure. In fact, this is why many sex therapists often recommend engaging activities that also stimulate a "feel-good" response, such as getting away for a romantic weekend, massage, or taking a bubble bath—they release dopamine. Unfortunately for many women, their dopamine response to these activities isn't strong enough because their underlying physiology isn't in balance. They need the dopamine equivalent of a double espresso. Fish oil is the key.

Fish oil has been shown in animal and human studies to raise dopamine levels in the brain. The active ingredient in fish oil is omega-3 fatty acid. There are two omega-3 fatty acids in fish oil: eicosapentaenoic acid, also known as EPA, and docosahexaenoic acid, called DHA. Though omega-3 fatty acids are most well known for reducing heart disease, lowering LDL (bad) cholesterol, raising HDL (good) cholesterol, slowing the fatty deposit buildup in the arteries, and reducing blood inflammation, more and more scientific research is coming out every day showing the importance of these two omega-3 fatty acids for general health. One of the most active fish oil researchers is Dr. Joseph Hibbeln at the National Institutes of Health, who has shown that fish oil improves cardiovascular health, reduces depression and aggression, and can aid in the treatment of bipolar disorder, among other things. He is a very vocal pioneer of fish oil supplementation and even has a meta-study examining cultures worldwide—showing how fish consumption is correlated with drops in many disease rates.

What does this have to do with dopamine and a woman's sexuality? A woman on the typical American diet is starving for dopamine, and dopamine is the key to female sexual pleasure. Dopamine is what makes a woman feel connected to her vulva, connected to feeling sensual, and able to experience touch. Dopamine makes things taste good, smell good, sound good, look good, and above all—feel good. How do you achieve a high level of dopamine? Take fish oil. Why fish oil, though? Why not just eat fish? And aren't there other things you can take to raise your levels of dopamine? Fish oil is just oil from fish, but honestly, are you going to eat fish every single night? And it has to be fatty fish, like salmon and tuna; the omega-3 fatty acids are in the fish fat. Fish that is fried is usually cooked in oils high in omega-6 fatty acids, canceling out the effect. Poached or grilled fish night after night would get old pretty quick, right? Not only that, it's not safe to eat fish daily anymore. Nowadays our oceans are so unclean that pollutants get right into the fish, and we end up eating them. Fish oil is refined and purified; toxic chemicals like mercury are removed, so it is safe to take fish oil every day. And easy, too.

Plenty of other things raise dopamine levels to some degree, including wild game, free-range beef and poultry, and shellfish. But the easiest, cheapest, and safest way to consume large amounts of EPA and DHA is through fish oil supplements.

Saturated and monounsaturated fats—found in meat, poultry, and dairy—will also raise dopamine levels somewhat, which is another reason many women today are at a dopamine disadvantage: so many of us are on low-fat diets. The fats found in dairy and some oils will increase your dopamine levels—and women tend to be psyched about that. "You mean, butter and ice cream are okay?" Sexually speaking, yes. Weight loss, now that's another matter, but there are good, balanced approaches to getting some fat in the diet and maintaining your weight—in fact some women even lose weight on the Orgasmic Diet. By relying more on proteins, reducing the amount of starchy carbs and sugars you eat, and avoiding trans fats and polyunsaturated fats, you can maintain or lose weight—but you'll read more on the eating aspect of the Orgasmic Diet later.

The Orgasmic Diet also recommends a moderate amount of dark chocolate. High-quality chocolate not only contains chemical compounds that increase dopamine levels, but it also has another that mimics the chemistry produced by being in love. Indeed, Italian researchers have shown that women who eat a small quantity of dark chocolate every day have better sex lives. Well, there's a case for eating chocolate!

But what about increasing my dopamine levels through pharmaceuticals, you may wonder. Can't I just go to my doctor and get a dopamine drug to boost my dopamine? Yes and no. Several clinical trials are being conducted right now on dopamine drugs to treat female sexual dysfunction. Pharmaceutical companies are looking at different approaches now that Viagra failed in clinical trials for women. But they haven't hit the market yet, and the companies are running into problems with getting the right dose; too much and the women start vomiting and fainting—two reactions we definitely don't want! Fish oil doesn't pose that problem.

Doctors are prescribing some off-label dopamine drugs right now to treat female sexual dysfunction, especially dysfunction brought on by antidepressant drugs; two include bromocriptine and ropinirole. Again, doctors are encountering dosing issues with the side effects of nausea and light-headedness, and often there is the disquieting problem of having to increase dosage over time to produce the same effect. Neither physicians nor women want to repeat what happened with an older dopamine drug, Survector (amineptine), which was used to treat depression and which caused spontaneous orgasms in some women; ultimately, it was pulled from the market because of substance abuse problems. Even some street drugs such as cocaine, heroin, and amphetamines are known to raise dopamine levels. My point? Dopamine isn't just a neurotransmitter of pleasure, it's the neurotransmitter of addiction.

In short, fish oil is a safe, healthy, and nonaddictive way to effectively raise dopamine levels and kick-start our ability to feel pleasure, especially sexual pleasure.

Serotonin: It's All About Balance

However, having enough dopamine in our bodies is just part of the solution to becoming turned on and orgasmic. The other major player in the biochemical puzzle is the neurotransmitter serotonin. Like dopamine, serotonin has many jobs in the brain: it enhances alertness, improves mood, and makes people feel happy and cheerful. High levels of serotonin help us handle stress, regulate appetite, and make us feel energized. Serotonin also affects sleep; when serotonin levels are low, we have trouble sleeping. And mightiest of all, low serotonin levels also cause us to feel depressed. In fact, almost all antidepressant drugs work by raising serotonin levels in the brain in one way or another.

This is how serotonin operates. Imagine you are Christmas shopping. You have a list, you are checking it twice. You know where all the sales are and the fastest way to get from store to store. As you flit from rack to display, your mind is racing, thinking over the recipient's tastes, anticipating the reaction on opening the present, remembering past gifts you have given. Working like clockwork, you buy the perfect present for everyone, in record time and on sale, and as you tick the names off your list you see you even have a little left over in your budget for a little something for yourself, so you get that perfect pair of shoes you've been wanting. You drive home and quickly reorganize your closets, finding hidden crannies to hide all the loot, packaging it up so it won't be noticed. As you are cooking dinner you're filled with satisfaction, but then your mind immediately jumps ahead to all the other Christmas items on your to-do list.

How do you feel right then? Your mind is buzzing with lists and organizational power and self-confidence and brisk industry. That is serotonin at work.

Our society is a very serotonin-oriented society. Women are expected to be high-functioning and efficient, to be organized and handle housework and children and jobs and a million and one things—to stay busy, busy, busy. Sometimes your serotonin just isn't there—the day looms, and your lengthy to-do list awaits you. And you just want to pull the covers over your head and go back to sleep. What do you do? You drink a cup of coffee. The mind is the brain and the brain is the mind. You instinctively know that coffee will give you that kick you need, that feeling of having just finished your Christmas shopping triumphantly, ready to move on to your next victory. And it works—you drink that cup of coffee and your mind sharpens and you are ready to face the day. A number of things besides caffeine can give that lift to some degree—cigarettes, your morning bagel, some ginseng tea. And for women who really can't get out of bed and feel that life isn't worth living, there of course are antidepressants. Antidepressants raise serotonin levels better than anything; that's what they are designed to do.

But too much serotonin can be a bad thing, especially when it comes to getting in the mood for sex. There you are, reorganizing your closets, getting ready to hide away those Christmas presents, and your boyfriend or husband comes up behind you and starts nuzzling your neck. "Can't you see I'm busy!" No, he can't, not really. Men have the edge in so many ways, sexually speaking; for example, they naturally have high levels of dopamine. So for a man it's generally pretty easy to step into that vacation-in-the-Bahamas frame of mind. Men just need to relax a bit. He's relaxed all right, coming up to you with his arms around you, but your mind is buzzing with ten thousand things you need to get done today. All of your focus is in your head; you feel his arms around you but you don't really *feel* his arms around you. That's the serotonin talking. To be in a sexual mood, you have to shut up that serotonin. What are you going to do, tear up your to-do list?

Sex therapists often do recommend a separation from the day's activities and the beginning of a relaxing evening as a way to help your mind and body relax. And for women with good and natural neurotransmitter function, this sort of ritual downtime is very effective. But what about those three lattes you drank to get through your day? Your body and mind are buzzing, and a simple meditation ritual or hot bath is not going to make all that caffeine instantly vanish from your body. You are stuck in a high-serotonin state, until eventually your serotonin crashes down when the coffee wears off, later that night when you're asleep.

And what about the woman on antidepressants who has a chemically induced, artificially high level of serotonin round the clock, seven days a week? Women on antidepressants have a very high incidence of drastically lowered libido and orgasmic ability. Antidepressants work so well in inhibiting sexuality they are even prescribed to men with premature ejaculation. Yes, they work well to boost your serotonin so you don't feel depressed, but they also take away your ability to feel sexual pleasure. (There is one exception, though, and that is Wellbutrin, an antidepressant that raises levels of both dopamine and serotonin at the same time.)

Obviously it would be a bad idea to have rock-bottom serotonin levels; very low serotonin levels cause depression. No one wants to be depressed, and depressed people usually don't want sex. Have steady, moderate serotonin levels as the goal, along with very high dopamine levels. That is the optimal state to get a woman's neurochemistry primed for enhanced sexuality with high libido and easy orgasms. It's a matter of balance.

If you can keep your dopamine levels high by consuming lots of fish oil, good dietary fat, and small amounts of chocolate every day, how can you keep your serotonin levels moderate and steady? There's a simple answer to that: avoid substances that spike serotonin or keep it too high. Activities that raise serotonin levels only do so temporarily. But you can get stuck with the serotonin from things you eat and drink until it wears off, so don't eat or drink them, at least not right before you plan on having sex. Yes, this includes coffee. And tea and caffeinated soda and even chocolate, if you eat too much. Chocolate contains some caffeine, so limit yourself to half an ounce of good dark chocolate a day. Smoking spikes serotonin (and it constricts blood vessels, also bad for sexual function). Even certain foods spike serotonin. Dr. Judith Wurtman at MIT has done extensive research showing the effect of carbohydrates on serotonin levels in the brain. By eating a meal of only carbohydrates with no protein or fat, you can very effectively spike neural serotonin levels, especially with quickly digested carbohydrates like pasta, bread, potatoes, and white rice.

As you will soon see, there are several ways to help achieve moderate serotonin levels, such as avoiding caffeine and other stimulants and staying away from sugary and starchy carbohydrates, including the recommendation that all meals have a 40-30-30 percent balance of carbohydrates, fat, and protein; the carbohydrates recommended are nonstarchy fruits and vegetables, which regulate serotonin in the brain at a moderate, steady level. More on that later!

Free Testosterone: The Tiger in Your Tank

So you have a high level of dopamine and moderate serotonin levels; is that all a woman needs to increase her libido and improve her sexual responsiveness? No; neurotransmitter balance is only the first of three things that control female sexuality from a physiological point of view. A woman with only the right neurotransmitter balance and nothing else will just want to do yoga and enjoy that spa retreat. Who needs a sex partner? Pure pleasure doesn't necessarily mean sexual pleasure. High dopamine levels may connect you to the sexual sensations between your legs, but if desire isn't there, what's the point?

Desire is complicated, especially in women. Women desire many things from their sex partner. We like to feel sexually attractive, we like the physical affection and intimacy from being held close, we like to feel our sexual power over men, we like to be romanced and seduced, of course we like to feel love, and yes, we even like that feeling of opening up a tiny box and seeing something sparkling and expensive inside. All of those things contribute to the multifaceted gem that is female desire. But the heart of the gem, where fire burns deep, is when you look into a man's eyes and he grabs you with his gaze and you feel his desire for you knife through you, kindling an immediate, burning need. You feel that need course through your body and provoke hunger to have him inside you right that instant! Now! And you look at his body, up and down and especially in the middle, and it's all you can do to stop yourself from pressing up against him hard right there in public and kissing him passionately.

That desire is caused by free testosterone, a form of testosterone. Free testosterone is determined by the ratio between the total level of testosterone in your body and the level of sex-hormone-binding globulin (SHBG) present. How much of that total testosterone gets freed up to become free testosterone is determined by the level of SHBG; the lower the SHBG, the higher the free testosterone. And it's the free testosterone that governs a woman's drive, at least physiologically speaking.

Some women never feel the effects of free testosterone. If you are one of those women who has never felt it, my diet may not be enough. You may also need to see an endocrinologist and have your testosterone levels checked. (You will find more about this topic later in the chapter on hormones.) But most women do have the potential for optimal hormonal functioning, sexually speaking. You just have to hit the right groove, and my diet will help you do that.

First a little background about testosterone is necessary. Everyone makes jokes about testosterone. Testosterone means male—

irritatingly male. Doesn't it? Not quite. Women's bodies make testosterone, too, in the ovaries and adrenal glands—much less than men's do, but the hormone is there (men's bodies make estrogen, too, in low levels). Just like men, as a woman ages, her body makes less testosterone. There are a number of things besides age that affect free testosterone levels in women—birth control pills, diet, exercise—with the result that many young women nowadays have the free testosterone levels of elderly women.

In their excellent book *For Women Only,* Dr. Jennifer Berman and Dr. Laura Berman say flat out, "To us, testosterone is so central to a woman's sexual function that no lover and no amount of sexual stimulation can make up for its absence. We have had significant success in treating our patients with testosterone and think it has a definite benefit for women with low desire and documented low testosterone levels."

Quite simply, free testosterone puts a tiger in your tank—it makes you think of men, sex, orgasms. You notice how men (or women) smell, how they look, how wonderful their bodies are. Free testosterone makes a woman's clitoris get hard easier and makes her have stronger orgasms. It makes you want more orgasms. Even women with normal levels of free testosterone will notice an increase in these areas if their free testosterone increases to robust levels. Not only does testosterone improve sex, it improves energy and the ability to build muscle mass. The more muscle a woman has, the easier it is for her to lose weight and look good. A healthy, substantial level of testosterone is not going to make you look like a bodybuilder or get hairy—it will simply make you a better you, and a more sexual you.

Most experts agree on the importance of testosterone. The Princeton Consensus Statement evaluated peer-reviewed literature and a consensus conference of international FSD experts and defined androgen insufficiency (low testosterone) in women. In particular this study focused on androgen insufficiency's bad effect on female sexuality, recommending treatment with testosterone replacement therapy (TRT) for women with low free testosterone levels. More directly, Dr. Andre Guay, a leading expert on FSD, has done a survey of women with a healthy sex drive and women with sexual dysfunction, showing the difference in free testosterone and other androgens. He found that women with healthy sexual functioning have higher free testosterone.

It should be no surprise that there have been studies questioning this finding—free testosterone is only one of three things that physiologically affect a woman's sexuality. There has also been a backlash from some experts who feel that too much focus has been given to testosterone, in particular on using TRT. My beliefs fall firmly on the side of the majority of doctors in this field who do believe free testosterone is a critical factor for female sexual function. I also believe a natural holistic way to improve free testosterone is the best path for most women to try first, before TRT.

And the fact remains: low free testosterone is associated with lack of desire, lack of sexual pleasure, and inability to orgasm—when a woman's free testosterone is very low she almost forgets what sex is all about. So how do you raise free testosterone?

First, you want a robust level of total testosterone. How do you get it naturally? Putting on muscle will help, but that takes time and a lot of work. The easier way is by eating monounsaturated and saturated fats. If your total testosterone is still low after increasing your fats, adding muscle tone may be necessary, and if that doesn't work, TRT might be necessary (see chapter 11 for further information on TRT). Nothing in the Orgasmic Diet will make your testosterone too high, so don't worry. What you're really trying to do is increase your total testosterone while keeping your SHBG at a low, healthy minimum. SHBG is needed by the body to bind with testosterone in order to regulate it. The problem occurs when, in response to our modern diet that is high in starchy carbs and sugar, as well as the impact of hormonal birth control pills, SHBG binds up more of the testosterone than it should. And when testosterone is bound up with SHBG, it is not available (i.e., free) to improve libido. Therefore, by keeping SHBG low and testosterone high, the body can use the testosterone to its best advantage.

On the Orgasmic Diet, SHBG is attacked from three different angles. If you can, change your birth control method to a nonhormonal form. Hormonal birth control raises SHBG. Eating the right balance of foods also keeps SHBG low, in particular eating protein at every meal and cutting back on carbohydrates. Finally, getting the RDA of zinc and magnesium in a basic over-the-counter vitamin supplement helps keep SHBG low (but because zinc and magnesium interfere with calcium, I also recommend getting the RDA of calcium at the same time for general health reasons).

Having low SHBG means your body enjoys more of the testosterone it has, and you feel desire, and your own body's sexual hunger. You want orgasms, and the longer you've been without one, the more you want one.

PC Muscle Tone and Good Genital Circulation

With a good level of free testosterone, you will feel desire; with high levels of dopamine and moderate levels of serotonin, you will be able to feel sensual pleasure; but you also must be able—literally— to feel sensual pleasure. So the final step for women whose quest is to enhance their libido and sexual responsiveness is to improve sensation and performance, and this means strengthening and toning your sex muscles and improving the circulation that brings sensitivity to your genitals.

Men generally have it easier than women when it comes to dopamine and testosterone levels; but men are sometimes overwhelmingly concerned with performance and experience difficulties for these reasons. But performance ability is important for women, too. While women may not need rock-hard clitorises to be able to enjoy sex, we do need our clitorises to be able to get hard. We need our vaginal tissues to be able to become engorged and swollen. Those things are determined by blood circulation to the genitals.

There are lots of things that improve blood circulation to the genitals, and men have used them all, sometimes all at once. Generally, those male "aphrodisiacs," herbs and other substances, don't just improve circulation, they often change neurotransmitter balance, frequently raising serotonin levels. For men, this is a bonus. Not only do they get a harder erection, they get a longer-lasting erection—and the substance is inducted into the male aphrodisiac hall of fame. For women this is a serious drawback. Women generally need to speed up their orgasms, not slow them down, and clitoral erection quality is always going to take a backseat to speed. So our options for improving genital circulation are much more limited.

This is where fish oil comes in—again. Fish oil is not only good at boosting dopamine, it also improves overall circulation—in fact, it is so effective in this respect that it is endorsed by the American Heart Association. Another way to improve circulation to any area of the body is to build up muscle in that body part. Most women have heard of Kegels, exercises that improve muscle tone in the vagina. Kegels exercise the PC muscles (pubococcygeus muscles).

First you must learn where the muscles are and what they feel like when they are flexed and relaxed. Then you must flex them regularly during exercise sessions.

Unfortunately, Kegels alone are not entirely effective for delivering sexual tone. A good analogy would be curling your arms up and down to build up bicep strength. Such an exercise would be useful for weak invalids, but the average person wouldn't see much of a benefit. Kegels are good for women who have recently given birth or women struggling with incontinence issues, but for most women even doing Kegels religiously will not yield the very strong PC muscles the Orgasmic Diet recommends. The way to build superior muscle tone is through resistance.

So how do you exercise your PC muscles with resistance? You use a resistance device. I reviewed most of the affordable PC muscle exercisers on the market for the Women's Sexual Health Foundation (www.twshf.com), comparing performance, effectiveness, and ease of use, including the GyneFlex, vaginal cone weights, the Kegelcisor, and the Kegelmaster 2000. I found that the best device is the GyneFlex, which I describe as a teeny, tiny Thighmaster that you insert in your vagina. Exercising with the GyneFlex device will give you superior PC muscle tone, much faster than you could hope for by doing Kegels alone. (You will find all there is to know about the GyneFlex and other Kegel devices in chapter 7.)

The benefits that come from having very strong PC muscles are more than just improved genital circulation. In her 1981 study with Dr. John D. Perry, "If Your Sexual Response Is Poor, the Cause Could Be Weak PC Muscles," published in the *International Journal of Human Relations,* renowned sex researcher and author Dr. Beverly Whipple showed that strong PC muscle tone is directly correlated to vaginal orgasmic ability. In addition, Dr. René Masse reported experimental proof in a paper presented at the Society for

Scientific Study of Sex in New York, November 1981, that Kegel exercises improved sexual arousal in women. He referred to "the first controlled experimental study supporting the theory that myotonia precedes vasocongestion," and said that "women assigned to Kegel exercise group had significantly higher sexual arousal (vasocongestion) than controls."

In other words, rather than having women subjectively rate their arousal and orgasms before and after improving PC muscle tone with Kegels, Dr. Masse measured the arousal with scientific instruments. It's a fact—PC muscle tone helps sexual arousal.

Of course, excellent PC muscle tone has the added benefit of giving a woman a tighter vagina, something both women and their partners can appreciate.

Excellent PC muscle tone also indirectly helps clitoral orgasms by improving circulation and stimulating the further end of the clitoris. Indeed, recent medical discoveries have shown the clitoris is much larger than previously thought, with the nerve network extending all the way back to the G-spot. So doing Kegels—with or without a resistance device—will indeed make clitoral orgasms sharper and more intense. (In chapter 9, you will find much more about clitoral orgasms—how to have one if you're currently unable to and how to make those you are having more intense, long-lasting, and pleasurable.)

However, the most direct benefit of excellent PC muscle tone is vaginal orgasms. If you are already vaginally orgasmic, improving vaginal muscle tone will make your vaginal orgasms stronger. If you are not yet vaginally orgasmic, exercising your PC muscles on their own wouldn't necessarily mean you would gain vaginally orgasmic ability. However, having very strong PC muscles, combined with the Orgasmic Diet, highly increases your odds of gaining the ability to have vaginal orgasms. With practice and by staying on the diet, you may even develop the ability to have spontaneous vaginal orgasms simply by flexing the PC muscles. Some women on my diet have, including me.

Some women who go on the diet choose not to do the PC muscle exercises—with or without a device—and the diet still works; it does improve libido very well and, as mentioned, adds intensity of feeling to your clitoral orgasms. My diet is all about choice; you choose how far you want to go. But personally, I think women who don't take this last step and don't use the resistance device are missing out: The rewards are so tremendous and vaginal orgasmic ability makes sex so great—whether your aim is to experience a simultaneous orgasm with your partner or a vaginal orgasm on your own.

Even if you are not a science buff, you can see how the underlying science of the Orgasmic Diet is straightforward. Now that wasn't so bad, was it? Let's move on and get you started on the ride of your life!

A note on vaginal orgasms

Women can experience vaginal orgasms with or without a partner, with or without penetration. In other words, even women who are not sleeping with men can experience the tremendous wow of the vaginal orgasm from the PC muscle contractions alone or in tandem with G-spot stimulation, manually or with a toy such as a dildo.

the nuts and bolts of the diet

PART TWO

CHAPTER FOUR

The Magic of Fish Oil

By now you are probably wondering how you actually follow this diet. I promise, it really is a very simple, easy-to-live-with diet. On the Orgasmic Diet, you will do the following:

1. Take supplements (especially fish oil); a multivitamin; the RDA of calcium, magnesium, and zinc; and extra iron and vitamin C.

2. Eat foods that raise dopamine and testosterone levels and keep your serotonin levels steady. You will try to get a balance of 40 percent carbs, 30 percent protein, and 30 percent fats at every meal. You will focus on carbs like nonstarchy vegetables and fruits. You will learn to avoid trans fats and polyunsaturated fats, including vegetable oils such as corn oil, soybean oil, and safflower oil, that counteract the benefits of the omega-3 fatty acids, instead

eating monounsaturated fats like olive or canola oil or moderate amounts of saturated fats found in dairy and meat. And you will eat a half-ounce of quality dark chocolate every day.

3. Avoid things that interfere with sexual function, including caffeine, cigarettes, and other stimulants; hormonal birth control; and drinking alcohol to excess.

4. Exercise the PC muscles, using the GyneFlex or a similar device, and over time tone your muscles completely.

And that's it. The Orgasmic Diet does not include any prescription medications or exotic-sounding herbals. The diet is just four basic steps that synergistically work together in a healthy and natural way to return your body to the sexuality all women deserve. So let's first take a look at the supplements you will be taking.

Why Fish Oil?

So far, you may be thinking that my diet doesn't seem that unusual or different from many of the successful eating plans out there today. However, skeptics frequently post arguments online against the plan. The most common is that there are already plenty of people on similar eating plans, like the Zone, the South Beach Diet, or the Atkins Diet, and plenty of those people take vitamins, avoid coffee, and eat dark chocolate—some even take fish oil supplements because they're known to be good for your heart, immune system, and some chronic diseases. So why are we not seeing hordes of rampaging women roaming the streets?

These skeptics have a valid point—my diet is about returning the body back to its natural healthy state, and in that way it's not entirely original or provocative. Aside from the PC muscle exercises that are part of my plan, the food portion of the diet is all about setting the stage, helping hormone levels become normal and healthy, and getting your brain in the best state for great sexual response. (And I would be willing to bet that women who are already on programs that echo these elements of the Orgasmic Diet enjoy a higher than normal sexual response.) These factors create the base upon which the true key to the diet rests: the fish oil. The fish oil is what truly sets my diet apart from other diets, because the dosage I recommend is very high. The extremely high level of fish oil I recommend is very unusual. If you are already taking fish oil—perhaps for your joints or your heart—I guarantee you are not taking even half the dose I recommend. I am recommending women take very, very high doses of fish oil—skyhigh levels, even. (You will see just how high in the next several pages.)

I am also advocating high-grade fish oil. The fish oil sold in drugstores is often low-grade. It is very diluted, containing lots of fish by-products mixed in with the active ingredient omega-3 fatty acids. Some women have told me that they would need to take over half of the entire bottle of capsules in one day to get the dose I recommend. Oy!

When I explain this detail to skeptics, they often find another angle to attack: "You are telling women to take fish oil like a medication. You aren't a doctor; isn't that dangerous?" Know that I do strongly recommend that before women start taking such a high dose of fish oil they check with their doctor, and in particular tell him or her just how high the dose of omega-3 fatty acids will be. Particularly, women on any kind of medication should check with their doctors before starting my plan. High-dose fish oil may interact with some medicines. (See page 62 for specific drug interactions to be wary of.)

Fish oil is not some exotic herb or new untried supplement; it's a natural element of the fish we eat, and humans have been eating fish as part of their diet for centuries. Although you could get the equivalent amount of omega-3 fatty acids I recommend from eating a large salmon steak for lunch and dinner every day, that would get dull pretty fast, and may even be dangerous due to mercury and other pollutants found in wild fish (and farm-raised fish have lower omega-3 fatty acid content). Because of this, it is not safe for a person to eat fish more than once or twice a week. The official recommendations from the FDA is to eat no more than up to fourteen ounces of fish that is low in mercury per week (three servings), while pregnant women, women who are planning to get pregnant, or nursing women should minimize their exposure to methyl mer-

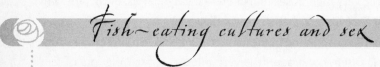

Fish—eating cultures and sex

In many cultures, a fish-centric diet is very common. For example, in Scandinavian countries fish has traditionally been such a common dish that at the turn of the century hired help would often complain about the never-ending menu of salmon to their superiors. And Scandinavian women do have a certain reputation for enjoying sex. Consumption of fish in Scandinavia has dropped in the modern era, but it is still high in Iceland. Coincidentally, in recent surveys of sexual habits worldwide conducted by the condom company Durex, Iceland held several world records. Iceland has the youngest average age of onset of sexual activity (15.7), the highest rate of vibrator ownership (52 percent), the highest likelihood of using sex toys (56 percent), the highest average number of sex partners (12.4), the highest rate of people who have one-night stands (71 percent), and the highest rate of population willing to see their taxes spent on contraceptives (56 percent). Now I'm not saying I think the Icelanders have it right, but I am saying that I think the large amount of omega-3 fatty acids consumed by these people has had a cultural influence, in particular in areas where women would stand out (for example, vibrator ownership). And by the way, my diet recommends Icelandic levels of fish oil!

cury by eating only twelve ounces per week (two servings of fish that is low in mercury). For further information on contaminants in fish visit www.epa.gov/waterscience/fishadvice.

On the other hand, high-grade fish oil supplements have the contaminants filtered out, so they become the best, safest, and most healthy way to consume omega-3 fatty acids.

A Secret Malnutrition

Skeptics also ask—why *fish* oil? Why is something so important to the survival of the human race—women's sexual pleasure—tied up with something so random and arbitrary? What about inland people? What about hunter-gatherers—did the women have low libidos? Wouldn't that be a serious evolutionary disadvantage? The answer to that, in my opinion, is yes. I firmly believe that women evolved to have a high libido and easy orgasmic function, at least in times of plentiful food. It makes evolutionary sense that a woman's desire would drop in times of famine; pregnancy requires a plentiful and constant food supply to ensure survival of the mother and her baby. But why do I focus on fish? The answer is that it wasn't just fish. Almost everything we ate as we were evolving was very high in omega-3 fatty acids. Grain didn't exist, except very rarely and in wild varieties. Fruit was also very rare, a seasonal treat (and was also much, much less sweet and calorie-dense than modern fruit). We evolved eating vegetables and critters. "Critters" is a loose category encompassing wild game, seafood, and even bugs. All these critters share something in common: in addition to being good sources of protein, they are all very high in omega-3 fatty acids.

So what happened? If wild game is high in omega-3 fatty acids, what happened to the cow and chicken? How come beef and poultry aren't high in omega-3 fatty acids? One word—cowboys. When we lost our cowboys, women lost their sex drive. Cowboys are more than just a sex symbol. Omega-3 fatty acid content is determined by what the animal ingests—you are what you eat. Cows that eat grass are high in omega-3 fatty acids, just like wild game, just like bison or buffalo. Grass-fed beef is chock-full of omega-3 fatty acids, and so is milk from the cows because the essential fatty acids are created in the cells of the green plants. Likewise free-range chickens that are not fed grain yield omega-3-fatty-acid-rich meat and eggs. The dead giveaway for food high in omega-3 fatty acids is a "gamey" taste. That gamey taste is good for you, just like the fishiness of fish.

This gets me back to cowboys, or rather their disappearance. Around the turn of the last century, modern farming methods changed drastically. No longer were cowboys working on the range, moving cattle from pasture to pasture. Instead, cattle and poultry were penned, caged, and fed a diet consisting almost completely of grains, instead of their natural diet primarily made up of grass. Cows and chickens that eat a grain-based diet yield meat, milk, and eggs high in omega-6 fatty acids. Omega-6 is produced in the seeds of plants; omega-3 is the leaves. Both fatty acids are essential, but too much omega-6 fatty acid can contribute to heart disease and other chronic conditions. Also, omega-6 fatty acids interfere with the libido-enhancing, heart healthiness of omega-3 fatty acids at the cell membrane level. So not only is the modern North American diet very low in omega-3 fatty acids, it is very high in omega-6 fatty acids. It's this imbalance in the ratio of omega-3 to omega-6 fatty acids that interferes with the proper functioning of omega-3 fatty acids. For the last hundred years this has resulted in a secret malnutrition in Western society.

At the turn of the last century heart disease wasn't as prevalent as it is now. Lots of other modern diseases were quite rare before the twentieth century, and it wasn't just because everybody died young of infectious disease. We were actually healthier back then. Indeed, in 1900, the top three causes of death in the United States were pneumonia and influenza, tuberculosis, and diarrhea/enteritis, with heart disease ranked as the fourth-leading cause of death. But by the 1970s, heart disease rose to the number one cause of death in the United States. And some scientists surmise that many modern diseases may simply be symptoms of an underlying omega-3 fatty acid malnutrition. In the last ten years, a tremendous amount of research is being done around the world investigating the amazing health benefits of taking omega-3 fatty acids. Omega-3 fatty acids have been shown to help with heart disease, inflammation, some cancers, depression, schizophrenia, ADD, bipolar disorder, dementia, hypertension, diabetes, asthma, psoriasis, emphysema, cystic fibrosis, irritable bowel syndrome, Crohn's disease, colitis, rheumatoid arthritis, and even menstrual cramps. (For references to studies and other support showing the health benefit of grass-fed meat, milk, and eggs, see www.eatwild.com.) I know it makes omega-3-rich fish oil sound like a panacea, like snake oil even, but this is what current research is revealing. (A great source for specific research on the benefits of omega-3 fatty acids is www.oilofpisces. com—I know the name sounds rather "woo woo," but it offers very up-to-date, well-researched sources.)

Certainly the body considers omega-3 fatty acids to be very valuable. The omega-3 fatty acid DHA is critical for fetal brain development. When a woman is pregnant, her body releases its stores of omega-3 fatty acids to her baby. As she nurses her baby, her body is further depleted; breast milk is also high in omega-3 fatty acids. Semen is also high in omega-3 fatty acids, which are absorbed by the vaginal walls. From this vantage point, you can say that omega-3 fatty acids act as an evolutionary currency. Omega-3 fatty acids are critical for the health of brain and body, and people on a Western diet are starving for them. Our bodies think we are struggling through a time of famine, so of course women don't want to have sex. Our bodies are telling us not to! The good news is that this malnutrition is easily reversed by simply following a different diet and taking a pill. Okay, a lot of pills, or actually capsules to be exact.

Reversing Your Sexual Malnutrition

So, how much fish oil do you take? Well, that depends on your weight and height. (And remember, before beginning to take fish oil supplements you should check with your doctor.)

Warning when using fish oil

Fish oil interacts with other medications in a similar way as aspirin. Both aspirin and fish oil are anti-inflammatory substances and thin the blood; therefore, they may interact negatively with pharmaceutical drugs in similar ways. So it is best to avoid taking fish oil if one is taking a drug that negatively interacts with aspirin. Blood-thinning medications like Coumadin, some hypertension medications, and some other over-the-counter pain relievers also interact with fish oil. Also do not take fish oil if you are scheduled for surgery, are allergic to seafood (of course), or have a defibrillator. This is just a general list; check with your doctor for interaction information for particular medications you may be taking. Fish oil thins the blood and this is where the risks generally lie.

If you are taking high-dose fish oil and you get a small cut and notice that it bleeds for longer than normal, you should cut back on your fish oil dosage. In general this is not a problem, even at very high doses, but some people can be sensitive. In rare cases, some people develop compulsive gambling habits and/or spending issues due to the high dopamine levels they achieve from taking dopamine drugs. This may theoretically happen with taking high-dose fish oil, but every person's body is different.

How I Followed the Orgasmic Diet

"Each day I take six omega-3 soft gels (EPA 400 mg, DHA 200 mg), one Evening Primrose Oil soft gel (1300 mg), one iron capsule (50 mg), one calcium/magnesium/zinc capsule (1000 mg Ca, 500 mg Mg, 100 mg Zn), one Ester-C (500 mg), two to four ounces of chocolate (70 percent cacao). I am more interested in sex, and in pleasing my man. I'm more relaxed and less inhibited—I also have easier orgasms."

—Martina

For a minute let's forget about specific brands of fish oil; I don't want to confuse things right now. Simply look at the label. American labeling requirements force companies to put exact amounts of EPA and DHA per capsule on every bottle. Be sure to see how many capsules the label mentions "per dosage;" some brands confusingly list the amount of EPA and DHA for two or even three capsules.

As noted in chapter 3, EPA stands for eicosapentaenoic acid (and I don't plan on spelling that one again). I will just call it EPA. Likewise, DHA is docosahexaenoic acid. These are the two omega-3 fatty acids you need on my diet. Every bottle of fish oil capsules will have these two ingredients listed on the label so you can ignore everything else—the important thing is to get a high amount of both. How high? Well, I think I have braced you enough. For a woman who is five feet, five inches and weighs 130 pounds, I recommend 1700 mg of EPA and 1300 mg of DHA per day. That is *a lot* of fish oil for a woman that size. A larger woman, who is five feet, ten inches and 230 pounds, can get away with much more, up to double that amount. These amounts are approximate so don't worry if your particular brand doesn't come out with an exact ratio of EPA to DHA. On average one capsule of ultrarefined fish oil contains 300 mg of EPA and 200 mg of DHA. The important thing is not to go over the amount for your weight and size, because, as I said, I am recommending *a lot* of fish oil. In fact, when taking this much fish oil a woman shouldn't eat fish more than once a week. Overdosing on fish oil can lead to a risk of hemorrhage, because of the blood-thinning properties of fish oil, so be careful. Here is my dosage, in rough table form:

Weight	EPA	DHA
130 pounds	1700 mg	1300 mg
170 pounds	2500 mg	2000 mg
230 pounds	3400 mg	2600 mg

Again, these are very rough estimates. Go by weight when you are considering dose. If a woman wants to be sexual at certain times, she should take the EPA and DHA separately; some brands are one or the other. Save up the DHA for the day and take it instead in the evening. Do not take more fish oil in one day than recommended. And do not save it up over a few days and take it all at once. If you want to cut back sexually, cut back on the DHA, which is the more fast-acting component.

Some Common Questions About Fish Oil

"Good God, you must be joking! Do I really need to take that much fish oil?" Sticker shock can be considerable. Fish oil is not cheap. But cheaper brands tend to have lower EPA and DHA concentrations so you have to take more. I do recommend the more

expensive ultrarefined brands like Sears/Carlson, Minami, Zone Labs Omega-Rx, and the GNC brand Concentrated Fish Body Oils for three reasons: they are very concentrated so you will need to take fewer pills, they are very refined so contaminants like mercury have been more thoroughly filtered out, and they tend to be much easier on the digestive system. Lower-grade fish oils tend to have more fish by-products that can cause side effects like fishy burps and indigestion. The key, to me, is to get more than 500 mg of EPA+DHA per one 1g capsule. The cost depends on dosage. A woman on the 1700 mg EPA 1300 mg DHA daily dose might end up spending about fifty dollars a month, which is a lot, but worth it. Another thing to keep in mind is that no matter what brand of fish oil you take, it will certainly keep you regular.

"How do you determine if a brand is refined?" A good rule of thumb is that each 1 g capsule should contain more than 500 mg of EPA and DHA combined. Some women on my diet have found a relatively ultrarefined inexpensive brand at Costco. Check the label and figure out the concentration for your particular brand.

"What about salmon oil? Is that better?" Fish oil with a particular fish in the name tends to be the lowest grade of fish oil. It is best to buy brands labeled with the generic term "fish oil."

"What about cod liver oil? Cod liver oil has EPA and DHA." You should *not* take cod liver oil in high doses. Cod liver oil is *not* on my diet. Cod liver oil not only contains EPA and DHA but also contains vitamins A and D. Taking very high doses of vitamins A and D can lead to vitamin toxicity.

"I'm a vegetarian; what about flaxseed or flaxseed oil?" Unlike cod liver oil, flaxseed oil can be taken in high doses. Just not high

enough. Flaxseed contains the omega-3 fatty acid ALA. Although it is an omega-3 fatty acid, ALA acts as a precursor to EPA and DHA and therefore needs to be converted into EPA and DHA in order to be usable. Unfortunately, the conversion ratio is ridiculous; in other words, you would have to drink gallons of flaxseed oil to get enough ALA to convert over to the dosage of EPA and DHA required. It isn't physically possible. However, there is another alternative for vegetarians. DHA comes from algae, and there is a plant-based DHA capsule called Omega Zen-3 with 300 mg of DHA per capsule. It's not a perfect fit, but since DHA does help libido more than the EPA, vegetarians will see benefits if they choose this route.

"What brand do you take?" I have tried a combination of the Sears/Carlson as well as Minami and the GNC brand. They all work about the same, with the Minami being slightly superior in my opinion.

"How do I take the fish oil?" Make sure to take it with food. Fish oil is hard on the digestive system and hard to take on an empty stomach. Also, when you begin taking fish oil, start out slowly. I generally recommend starting off with one capsule a day, increasing to two capsules a day after a week, and so on, adding a capsule each week until you reach the full dosage for your height and weight. And trust your body; if you reach a threshold where you are having negative effects, such as gas or diarrhea, do not increase the dosage further (and check with your doctor). Spread your fish oil consumption throughout the day; if you are taking six capsules, for example, take two at breakfast, two at lunch, and two at dinner.

"Where do I find the fish oil?" The easiest way to buy fish oil, particularly ultrarefined fish oil, is online. Generally, if you find a

brand you like, you can create a standing order, charged to your credit card every month. Then your supply magically appears in the mail every month when you need it. If you prefer to go shopping, I recommend specialty supplement stores like the Vitamin Shoppe or GNC. Regular drugstores tend to carry only the lowest grade of fish oil. As I mentioned above, sometimes you may also find very good deals on ultrarefined fish oil at stores like Costco.

"Can I take fish oil while I am pregnant or nursing?" Yes, you can and you actually should. DHA is critical for infant brain development. I started taking fish oil when I was pregnant on the advice of my natal nutritionist. Of course, check with your obstetrician and your natal nutritionist (if you have one) before starting any new supplement. However, if you do take fish oil while pregnant or nursing, it is very important that you take only the purest and most ultrarefined brand. This is not the time to cut costs. I would say only take the Minami or Zone Labs Omega-Rx brand while you are pregnant or nursing. If you are taking a prenatal vitamin that contains fish oil, make sure you don't take an excessive amount of additional fish oil.

"I suffer from depression and am taking antidepressants. I see you mention research has been done on fish oil and depression. My antidepressants are interfering with my libido and orgasmic function. So will fish oil help me?" For women who are on antidepressants I strongly recommend a good ultrarefined brand, and to also attempt to take the full dosage of fish oil appropriate to your height and weight. Fish oil does help many women with depression and you may find after taking it for several months that you can decrease your antidepressant dose, under the supervision of your doctor.

"Will I smell like fish if I take this much fish oil?" It depends on the fish oil brand you are taking. This is another reason for taking ultrarefined fish oil—this side effect will not occur.

"What does the fish oil do, sexually speaking?" Fish oil both increases nitric oxide in your bloodstream, similar to Viagra, and increases dopamine levels in the brain, increasing feelings of pleasure and enhancing sensation.

"Can I get addicted to fish oil?" Only in the way that you can get addicted to vitamin C. Your body needs omega-3 fatty acids, just like vitamin C. If you go off the fish oil, you will be returned to the state you were in before you started taking the fish oil.

"Will the fish oil change anything besides my libido and orgasms?" Yes, absolutely. It will increase your feelings of pleasure and well-being in general. And you may notice an improvement in your health, even your mental health. Women who take high-dose fish oil generally have softer, younger-looking skin. Your skin becomes dewy and perhaps a little oily. Hair will be shinier and healthy, though it can become more oily, too; you won't be able to skip a day washing your hair. I can generally tell just from looking at a woman if she has been on my diet a month. Something I have found through my own experience is that I have to be careful listening to music because it sounds so wonderful, my tendency is to turn it up too loud. Finally, fish oil does something peculiar to one's eye color. It's not so much that it has changed my eye color, but it has made the irises more light-reflecting and dewy. This sounds odd, I know.

"Is there a downside to taking fish oil? Do I need to be careful?" Yes, you should be careful not to exceed the dosage since these recommendations are at the higher limit of safety. Also, fish

oil oxidizes very easily. When it does, it begins to smell a little spoiled. It is important to keep it out of direct heat and light. Keep the bottle capped and away from any radiators to avoid the risk of oxidization. In any case, it is very important to take antioxidants while taking fish oil to combat the oxidizing effects of the fish oil in the body. A good multivitamin should contain these antioxidants and should certainly be taken every day, along with fruits, vegetables, and dark chocolate.

"Are there any other side effects to taking fish oil?" Some people experience fishy burps, gas, slight indigestion (which is why I recommend taking your fish oil with a meal), and diarrhea.

Other Supplements

Most of this chapter has been about the dosage of fish oil recommended on my diet, because it is extreme and unusual. The rest of the supplements I recommend, while also important to get your sexuality perfectly in tune, are much less controversial. As I just mentioned, a multivitamin is important not just for general health, but also to counteract any potential fish oil that has oxidized. I also recommend extra vitamin C, and for those women still menstruating, extra iron. Women tend to not get enough of these vitamins in their diet. For the extra vitamin C, a glass of orange juice a day is enough, although you can certainly take a vitamin C supplement if you prefer. The iron is also helpful, and it is unlikely that constipation will occur from taking iron while taking high-dose fish oil. I recommend a very low dose of iron above that found in a multivitamin; you may need to get a pill-cutter, or take a low-dose iron pill every other day or every third day. It is not an exact science. Women who have stopped menstruating shouldn't take extra iron, and of course women who have the condition hemochromatosis shouldn't take iron at all. Hemochromatosis is latent in a large percentage of the population; check with your doctor before taking the iron.

I suggest the recommended daily allowance of calcium/magnesium/zinc. Generally this means a woman will be taking more than the RDA of zinc because most multivitamins also contain zinc. That's okay (unless you are very petite, in which case you may want to check with your doctor). Zinc and magnesium help keep SHBG low and free testosterone high. Generally it is best to spread out the calcium/magnesium/zinc pills throughout the day, and away from the morning multivitamin. If you take all three of the calcium/magnesium/zinc pills at once, your body won't be able to absorb all of the minerals.

As an overview, here is what you will be taking on the Orgasmic Diet:

Every Day

* Fish oil, containing approximately 1700 mg EPA, 1300 DHA
  (see instructions on page 64 for estimating amount right for you)
* The RDA of calcium/magnesium/zinc (1000/400/15 mg)
* A good multivitamin
* Extra vitamin C (a glass of orange juice a day is enough)

Every Two or Three Days

* 27 mg of iron

These vitamin and mineral recommendations are very straightforward and close to the RDA.

I know this is a lot of pills, but I think you will find that the results will be worthwhile. The following lists show a typical schedule for a woman taking all of the supplements I recommend, spread out throughout the week.

Sunday

- ❏ Multivitamin
- ❏ Vitamin C (or orange juice)
- ❏ Morning fish oil (two pills)
- ❏ Afternoon calcium/magnesium/zinc (two pills)
- ❏ Afternoon fish oil (two pills)
- ❏ Evening calcium/magnesium/zinc (one pill)
- ❏ Iron
- ❏ Dark chocolate (½ ounce)

Monday

- ❏ Multivitamin
- ❏ Vitamin C (or orange juice)
- ❏ Morning fish oil (two pills)
- ❏ Afternoon calcium/magnesium/zinc (two pills)
- ❏ Afternoon fish oil (two pills)
- ❏ Evening calcium/magnesium/zinc (one pill)
- ❏ Dark chocolate (½ ounce)

Tuesday

- ❏ Multivitamin
- ❏ Vitamin C (or orange juice)
- ❏ Morning fish oil (two pills)
- ❏ Afternoon calcium/magnesium/zinc (two pills)
- ❏ Afternoon fish oil (two pills)
- ❏ Evening calcium/magnesium/zinc (one pill)
- ❏ Iron
- ❏ Dark chocolate (½ ounce)

Wednesday

- ❏ Multivitamin
- ❏ Vitamin C (or orange juice)
- ❏ Morning fish oil (two pills)
- ❏ Afternoon calcium/magnesium/zinc (two pills)
- ❏ Afternoon fish oil (two pills)
- ❏ Evening calcium/magnesium/zinc (one pill)
- ❏ Dark chocolate (½ ounce)

Thursday

- Multivitamin
- Vitamin C (or orange juice)
- Morning fish oil(two pills)
- Afternoon calcium/ magnesium/zinc (two pills)
- Afternoon fish oil (two pills)
- Evening calcium/magnesium/ zinc (one pill)
- Iron
- Dark chocolate (½ ounce)

Friday

- Multivitamin
- Vitamin C (or orange juice)
- Morning fish oil (two pills)
- Afternoon calcium/ magnesium/zinc (two pills)
- Afternoon fish oil (two pills)
- Evening calcium/magnesium/ zinc (one pill)
- Dark chocolate (½ ounce)

Saturday

- Multivitamin
- Vitamin C (or orange juice)
- Morning fish oil (two pills)
- Afternoon calcium/ magnesium/zinc (two pills)
- Afternoon fish oil (two pills)
- Evening calcium/magnesium/ zinc (one pill)
- Dark chocolate (½ ounce)

The power of fish oil cannot be underestimated. As Dana, a thirty-something woman from Dallas shared with me, "As an experiment one weekend, I cut out eating fish, dropped the fish oil supplements completely, and drank regular Diet Coke instead of water or decaf Diet Coke. It took one day for my libido to evaporate. The speed of the change surprised me. A day later, I resumed the diet, and two days later my libido was back." Need I say more?

CHAPTER FIVE

This Is a Foodie Diet

Every day women are bombarded with yet one more diet promis- ing weight loss, happiness, and freedom from a preoccupation with food. Well, now it's time to relax. The Orgasmic Diet is not focused on weight loss, but rather on helping you become sexually energized, able to access your innate sexual desire and orgasm when and how you wish. You don't have to worry about calories. You don't have to weigh or measure servings, count points, or follow prescriptive recipes. All you have to do is eat a well-balanced, healthy diet with a great assortment of foods, many of which you are probably already eating and enjoying. As Lisa said, "For me, this was easy! It's really a healthy eating diet with a high protein content and less fatty and sugary foods!"

You will not gain weight on this diet, and who knows—you may even lose weight! Most women with whom I have spoken have either lost weight or maintained their weight. Why? Because the recommended ratio of protein, fat, and carbohydrates is best for your metabolism!

Essentially, the Orgasmic Diet is a high-protein, low-carb, "good-fat" diet, in which you try to achieve a 40/30/30 percentage balance. (Again, by "good fat" I mean a limited amount of monounsaturated and saturated fats, which raise dopamine levels and don't interfere with the Orgasmic Diet's increased consumption of omega-3 fatty acids.) This ratio of foods is similar in design and content to many current diets that promote this kind of balanced eating with an emphasis on whole foods The key with the Orgasmic Diet is to eat this way as part of the Orgasmic program.

On the Orgasmic Diet, you will essentially be eating:

✳ 30 percent protein, including meat, poultry, eggs, dairy, legumes, and occasional fish. Staying on a high-protein/low-carb diet will lower SHBG, which in turn will raise free testosterone. It is the free testosterone that controls a woman's sexual desire.

✳ 30 percent particular fats, specifically monounsaturated fats such as olive oil and saturated fats such as dairy, meat, and poultry. These particular fats will increase total testosterone and boost your libido and ability to orgasm.

✳ 40 percent or less carbohydrates, avoiding white breads, sugar, potatoes, and desserts. Lowering your consumption of starchy and sugary carbohydrates, and never making an entire meal of these foods, will also help you lower SHBG and avoid spikes in serotonin; remember, very high levels of serotonin are associated with a decrease in sexual functioning.

✻ As many fruits and vegetables as you wish; indeed, many women replace starchy carbs with carbs that are high in fiber, such as fruits and vegetables. These complex carbohydrates help maintain healthy serotonin levels—the sugar in fruit and vegetables is fructose, which takes longer to break down than processed sugar and is further slowed down by the fiber content—avoiding serotonin spikes.

✻ A half-ounce of dark chocolate per day, which will boost dopamine (the neurotransmitter enabling women to experience sexual pleasure).

You will be avoiding the following:

✻ Caffeine in all its forms (coffee, tea, and soft drinks), as caffeine spikes serotonin and interferes with a proper serotonin-dopamine balance.

✻ Trans or hydrogenated fats such as margarine and vegetable shortening and foods made with these substances (packaged baked goods, crackers, snacks). Trans fats are not only bad for your overall health but will counteract the dopamine-raising effect of the omega-3 fatty acids in the fish oil supplements you will be taking.

✻ Polyunsaturated fats, specifically corn, soybean, cottonseed, sunflower, and safflower oils, which are often found in packaged foods or called for in some recipes. These fats are made up mostly of omega-6 fatty acids, which will counteract the positive effect of the omega-3 fatty acids found in your fish oil supplements (as you saw in the last chapter, fish oil increases your libido and sexual responsiveness by increasing your levels of dopamine).

One of the beauties of this diet is that it's easy. It does not require a lot of planning, shopping, or preparing. It doesn't even require that much thinking. Once you get accustomed to balancing the various food groups and become familiar with what to leave out of your diet (most important, caffeine, starchy carbs, and polyunsaturated and trans fats), then choosing what to eat for breakfast, lunch, and dinner will be as easy as—having an orgasm!

Do you like chocolate? It's on the diet! Do you enjoy sushi? Steak? Cheese? They're on the diet. The Orgasmic Diet is both rich in taste and satisfying to eat. You will never feel hungry—well, except for the lover in your life!

Portion Sizes

Again, this isn't a weight-loss diet, so portion sizes are up to you. It's all about proportion. In general, the Orgasmic Diet recommends that all meals have a 40-30-30 percent balance of carbohydrates, protein, and fat. The carbohydrates recommended are nonstarchy fruits and vegetables, which promote moderate, steady levels of serotonin in the brain.

You're probably closer Than You Think

Many women hear the word *diet* and either freeze or freak. "A diet? Oh God, that means deprivation!" The Orgasmic Diet is not about deprivation—how could it be; it includes chocolate. Here are some questions to ask yourself:

1. Do I enjoy eating fruits and vegetables?

2. Do I like grilled chicken or meat?

3. Do I watch how often I eat sugary desserts or candy?

4. Am I already watching my intake of starchy bread and bagels?

If you answered yes to any of these questions, then you are more than halfway there! This is a diet filled with your favorite foods!

As a general rule of thumb, looking at all of the food on your plate, your meat or other protein source should take one quarter of the space, and the rest should be vegetables. If you are having rice or pasta or other starchy carbs, it should be no more than a quarter of the space, with another quarter being your protein and the other half of your plate being vegetables. These measurements also allow for an unseen but important space for fat—in the form of salad dressing, butter, or oil, and of course your daily chocolate fix!

And keep in mind, if you are eating a naturally high-fat cut of meat or if your protein is cheese or nuts, you don't need to add any extra fats (you will still be covering your omega-3s with your fish oil supplement). However, if your protein source is low-fat, then you will want to add fat to your vegetable, whether it be olive oil salad dressing or a bit of butter. Don't cut fat out of your diet completely; your libido needs fat.

Don't Be Afraid of Fats

The Orgasmic Diet does include fat; in fact, it relies on fat to work, as fat is what enables the body to maintain a healthy level of testosterone. And yet it's hard not to be afraid of fats when the media and the medical community have been bombarding us with the health

Eyeball your portions

If you prefer to eyeball proportions, think of portions as one fist of protein, one fist of starchy carbs, and two fists of vegetables, or three fists of vegetables. (Leave out the fats—either they are contained in the protein or the vegetables are cooked in them.) A deck of cards is also a good guideline for the size for protein at each meal.

All types of fat contain the same number of calories. On the Orgasmic Diet, you want one-third of your calories to come from fat. There are nine calories in one gram of fat, as opposed to typically four in low-fat protein.

And remember,
1 teaspoon of fat = 1 pat of butter = 4.5 grams of fat = 45 calories

risks caused by dietary fat. Let me put you at ease with some scientific facts about fat and your health.

It's commonly believed that saturated fats and dietary cholesterol "clog" arteries and cause heart disease. But as Stephen Byrnes, PhD, RNCP, points out in his article "Are Saturated Fats Really Dangerous for You?," a study known as the Framingham Heart Study is often cited as proof that dietary cholesterol and saturated fat are the root cause of heart disease. However, the study showed no correlation between how much saturated fat one ate and high cholesterol. In other words, it's the cholesterol that causes disease, not the saturated fat.

Byrnes goes on to say that on the contrary, "studies have shown that arterial plaque is primarily composed of unsaturated fats, particularly the polyunsaturated ones, and not the saturated fats of animals, palm, or coconut." In addition, it is trans fats that have been shown to be the true cause of atherosclerosis (clogging of the arteries), coronary heart disease, cancer, and other diseases.

Further, Byrnes points out that "studies have shown repeatedly that low-fat diets are associated with depression, cancer, fatigue, and violence," among other negative side effects. Here is a quick list of the benefits of eating saturated fats:

✳ They are rich in trace minerals such as selenium.

✳ They protect against cancer and fungal infections.

✳ They help the body utilize essential fatty acids.

✳ They lower blood levels of artery-damaging lipoproteins.

✳ They are necessary for proper calcium utilization in bones.

✳ They stimulate the immune system.

✳ They add structural stability to the cell and intestinal wall.

So, when eaten in moderation, saturated fats are a key part of good overall health.

Seven Days of Meals

Remember, it's easy to be on the Orgasmic Diet, so easy in fact that you won't feel like you're even on a diet. You will simply eat in this totally satisfying way. And you don't have to stress about being creative. You can follow my seven-day meal below and use it as a general guideline for how to eat.

Following is a sample seven-day meal plan with suggestions for breakfast, lunch, and dinner to get you started on the Orgasmic Diet, but as you will see, it's easy to create your own on-plan meals without too much advance work.

First a word about breakfast: Yes, breakfasts are hard on this diet, just as on any 40-30-30 diet. Since it is key to start out your day with sufficient protein, and because we tend to think of breakfast foods as based around breads and cereals, it's often challenging to be creative and inventive on this plan. I mostly eat eggs, eggs, eggs. If you are going to have extra carbs during the day, the best time is breakfast, unless you are planning on having sex right after. Do try to get some protein in your breakfast, even if you love buttered toast. Whatever your protein choice, round out your meal with a piece of fruit and/or some orange juice. And of course, eat a half-ounce of dark chocolate! I tend to eat mine at breakfast—what a great way to start the day!

Monday

Breakfast: Yogurt or cottage cheese, blueberries, strawberries, and granola.

Lunch: Chicken Caesar salad—grilled shredded chicken, romaine lettuce, shredded parmesan cheese, and Caesar dressing. You can add walnuts, pine nuts, olives, or grapes to add some flavor.

Dinner: Meatloaf, a side of green bean casserole, and salad.

Tuesday

Breakfast: Turkey sausage omelet with tomatoes, onions, and peppers.

Lunch: Vegetable quiche and fresh fruit.

Dinner: Chinese stir-fry in peanut oil with lean beef strips, red peppers, broccoli, onions, mushrooms, and bamboo shoots (I cheat and use frozen Chinese stir-fry vegetable mix and preprepared sauce in a bottle) and a small portion of white rice (about a half cup).

Wednesday

Breakfast: Two slices of bacon, one or two eggs, and a piece of toast.

Lunch: Cheeseburger (without the bun) and a big salad with everything—but no dressing.

Dinner: Greek chicken pitas with Greek yogurt sauce made with cucumber, onion, and garlic, and a salad of tomato, peppers, cucumber, Greek olives, feta, and olive oil.

Thursday

Breakfast: Yogurt topped with granola and fruit of your choice.

Lunch: Ham and swiss cheese on eight-grain bread with mayonnaise or mustard, pepper strips, and carrot sticks.

Dinner: Roasted chicken with a side of broccoli, and a salad with olive oil dressing.

Friday

Breakfast: Frittata with egg, onions, peppers, and Monterey cheese and salsa on top if you like it.

Lunch: Tuna nicoise salad—pan-seared tuna over greens, black olives, capers, hard-boiled egg, and crumbled blue cheese.

Dinner: Eggplant parmigiana and a bean salad.

Saturday

Breakfast: Scrambled eggs with cheese and bacon or sausage on the side.

Lunch: Twice-baked potato skin stuffed with chili, and cantaloupe or fruit salad.

Dinner: Steak fajitas and a side of sautéed onions and peppers and avocado with salsa to top.

Sunday

Breakfast: French toast, heavy on the egg.

Lunch: Pecan-grape chicken salad (diced chicken mixed with one teaspoon of mayonnaise, 1 tablespoon chopped pecans, 2 tablespoons chopped grapes) on a bed of greens.

Dinner: BBQ pork tenderloin, a side of broccoli, and a salad.

What Happened to Me on the Diet

"I started the diet because I was intrigued by the claim that it could start or increase orgasms, particularly the claim of becoming vaginally orgasmic, something I've never been. I don't anticipate ever going off the diet since it's a healthy diet, regardless of any orgasmic benefits it provides. Not only does it improve my sexual health but my overall health! It's very close to what nutritionists and physicians have been recommending with only a little bit of tinkering around the edges. I've even lost weight, which is great."

—Roberta

Tailoring the Diet to Your Wishes

Another fabulous feature of the Orgasmic Diet is learning and knowing that you can now control your own sexuality through what you eat and when. By being able to tailor the diet to meet your own needs and desires, you will not only feel more in charge of how and when you want to be and feel sexual but you will also feel more sexually confident. Some women like to feel sexual every day—they enjoy the blood pumping through their veins, the pulsing energy between their legs. The sexual heat inside of them makes them feel alive and radiant. As Connie said, "I like the way I feel—inside and out. I feel more sexually confident, and more attractive." Another woman, Gail, said, "I like the attention I get from men—in my car at the stop sign, in line at the supermarket, or walking down the street. It's as if men know!"

And if they have a man in their lives, these women like to meet their mate's desire head-on! As Carol explained, "I used to hate to feel pressure to be in the mood every time my husband wanted to have sex. Now I want to have sex—it's such a relief and pleasure to be in synch with him."

Some women prefer to take a day or two off from feeling sexual, or they prefer to feel sexual only at night. Jackie told me this about her experience: "I am a busy mom with three young kids. Most nights both my husband and I are flat-out exhausted. We don't have the energy for sex. But now we kind of plan it for the weekend nights. On those days and the day before, I increase my dose of fish oil, avoid caffeine, and watch my carbs. It's so easy! And boom— we're right there in the moment!"

Being on the Orgasmic Diet is all about you and how you want to feel. Your sexuality is under your control. Most women who are on the diet have told me that they didn't have to radically change the way they eat. They are simply more aware of how certain foods impact their libido and orgasmic ability. "If I binge on carbs and dessert, I not only feel down," twenty-nine-year old Marissa explained, "but I have no desire for sex. It's that simple. So now, when I know my boyfriend is coming over, I just don't eat those foods." Other women take a more rigid approach to the diet, knowing that if they even take one bite of a cookie, they will eat a whole box. Deanna, a thirtysomething administrative assistant from Wisconsin, said, "I can't go near sweet things or I will binge. So I just stay away—I feel better and I feel sexual—what could be better than that? And I don't even have a boyfriend at the moment!"

Take a look at the following descriptions. Use them as a guide to maximize your results, modify your results, or simply skip a day when you feel like it. Again, you can calibrate the diet to your liking, depending on how sexually intense you want to feel on any given day.

To Feel Sexual All Day

If your aim is to feel sexual all day long, you need to maximize those foods that increase dopamine and testosterone levels, stabilize serotonin levels, and improve genital circulation. So you will want to completely avoid caffeine and white sugar, limit your carbohydrates to fruit and vegetables, and focus on protein and fats such as olive or canola oil. You will also want to avoid or greatly limit alcohol.

Sample menu

Breakfast: Two eggs scrambled in butter, orange juice, and a half-ounce of quality dark chocolate.

Lunch: Big salad, heavy on the canola or olive oil dressing, and a slice of roast beef.

Snack: Fruit and nuts.

Dinner: If you are having a family dinner, just eat the meat and vegetables; avoid any starchy foods and desserts. Here's a fast dinner to prepare: Chop up some sirloin steak tips, add a bag of frozen mixed vegetables and a premixed sauce like teriyaki, and stir-fry in a skillet.

For Feeling Very Sexual Only at Night

If you are planning on having sex in the evening, then you can adjust the diet a bit, focusing on foods that increase dopamine levels and stabilize serotonin levels. You can have some caffeine early in the day. Continue to watch carbohydrates, especially white sugars, as they can cause a swing in serotonin. Rely on proteins, and avoid trans fats, which are always bad for you.

Sample menu

Breakfast: If you drink coffee or tea, now is the time. Have only one cup, and nothing very strong like espresso. Try oatmeal—old-fashioned oats cooked with salt, cinnamon, and brown sugar and mixed with regular-fat or low-fat vanilla yogurt; eat a half-ounce of good dark chocolate.

Lunch: Tuna sandwich (use whole-grain bread). Make with tuna packed in olive oil (is the nicest but expensive—regular tuna packed in water works, too), ~~canola~~ olive oil mayonnaise, and extras to taste—pickle relish, chopped celery, or whatever is preferred. Have finger vegetables— carrots, cucumbers, etc.—on the side.

Snack: Fruit and nuts.

Dinner: Moroccan chicken made with onions, garlic, olive oil, tomatoes, carrots, celery, zucchini, cinnamon, cumin, turmeric, saffron, salt, honey, and raisins. Have fruit for dessert—mango, fresh figs, dates, peaches, plums, pomegranate, strawberries, or pears—whatever is in season and looks appealing at the market. And a very small liqueur, two or three swallows to help relax you; any more would slow down your orgasm.

To Take a Day Off from Feeling Sexual

Many women like to take a day off from the diet, which enables them to drink caffeinated beverages and eat foods such as pasta and desserts. You don't need to watch your sugar or carbs as much, as their immediate impact on you sexually is not key.

Sample menu

Breakfast: Coffee or tea if you drink it (you can also have it later in the day), high-fiber whole-grain cereal with milk or whole-grain buttered toast with yogurt, and a half-ounce of good dark chocolate.

How They Followed the Orgasmic Diet

"My diet was already fairly high-protein and low-carb; I lost over thirty-five pounds over two years ago and have mostly kept it off this way. My main high-protein meal is usually breakfast. I find that eating my main serving of protein early in the morning leaves me less hungry and more energetic the rest of the day. I have my main carb serving in the middle of the day, and then try for a light supper. I discovered Lara bars and Cliff nectar bars, which are based on unsweetened dates instead of grains or soy, and I usually have one of those as a midmorning or midafternoon snack. The largest change for me has been eliminating soy products. Now I read labels carefully."

—Carol

"The first thing I did was cut out anything with caffeine. I've switched to drinking primarily water and decaf green tea with the occasional decaf diet soda. I seldom eat meat but I do try and eat fish once a day—for omega-3 and protein boost. I also drink two cups of low-cal cranberry juice and two cups of skim milk per day. I haven't acquired any chocolate yet but will get some soon. I've been boosting my intake of colorful veggies and fruits, including broccoli, cauliflower, snap peas, green beans, spinach, collard greens, mushrooms, bell peppers, and lots of berries. I also have one cup of low-fat yogurt each day."

—Roberta

Lunch: Hummus, and finger vegetables and crackers, pita, or breadsticks to dip in (check for trans fats, which can interfere with dopamine).

Snack: Cheese and fruit.

Dinner: Pasta supper with meat sauce (meatballs and sweet Italian sausage), a large salad with canola or olive oil dressing, and dessert if you like (but still stay away from trans fats).

Aphrodisiacs and Beyond

Most women who enjoy food and eating will be delighted by the foods they can eat on the Orgasmic Diet. And if you like to experiment with foods, you might be interested in some special foods that have been associated with increasing sexual desire or performance. For instance, did you know that Casanova only drank hot chocolate, not wine? Throughout history people have enjoyed chocolate to enhance sexual pleasure. And for as long as humans have created cultures, they have looked to food as potential sources of aphrodisiacs. Indeed, the website www.gourmetsleuth.com offers some very interesting history about the relationship between various foods and their sexual impact. Citing the *Cambridge World History of Food,* the Gourmet Sleuth points out that historically, "a distinction was made between a substance that increased fertility versus one that simply increased sex drive." Even the ancients seemed to understand that one of the reasons for a loss of libido and a decrease in fertility was the scarcity of certain foods. So by virtue of trial and error or some other magical thinking, people began making associations between various foods and their reproductive or sexual power.

Such associations were recorded as far back as the ancient Greeks of the first century A.D. and later by Paul of Aegina from the seventh century. The ancient list included anise, basil, carrot, salvia, gladiolus root, orchid bulbs, pistachio nuts, rocket (arugula), sage, sea fennel, turnips, skink flesh (a skink is a type of lizard), and river snails. The ancients suggested you steer clear of dill, lentil, lettuce, watercress, rue, and water lily. The ancients may not have had the scientific method, but they were very careful observers of the natural world and clearly understood cause and effect very well. Looking a little closer at this very interesting list, you can see the science glimmering underneath. For example, consider orchid bulbs. Orchid bulbs have for centuries been made into a drink called salep, popular in ancient Greece (when it was known as satyrion or priapiscus), the Middle East, and even England. This drink had a reputation as an aphrodisiac, in addition to being a general health tonic. Also, a species of orchid is the source for vanilla, a scent that can stimulate the libido in both men and women.

Another flower bulb with a sexual reputation is the iris. The secret aphrodisiac history of this flower stretches back through time. The emphasis on the flower, the fleur-de-lis, symbol of kings and prostitutes (and if you believe Dan Brown, the Priory of Sion), may point to the underlying secret of the iris root, also known as orris root, jezebel root, and Queen Elizabeth root. It is a very interesting plant with a very interesting history, intertwined with sex. People valued its beauty, but they valued the physiological effect on women of consuming the root more.

Sage is a type of salvia. Sage, a popular herb both at Thanksgiving and with new age practitioners, can actually be made into a very serious mind-altering drug. I am certain the ancients were aware of this, being masters of essential oils and perfumery. When sage is reduced to an essential oil, it must be handled with great care. Essential sage oil contains a high concentration of a toxic chemical called thujone. Thujone is found in absinthe. Large doses have many negative effects, ranging from nausea, vomiting, insomnia, restlessness, vertigo, tremors, and seizures, all the way up to delirium, convulsions, seizures, paralysis, brain damage, renal failure, and death. Though not something to experiment with, thujone does have an aphrodisiac reputation based on real chemistry. High levels of GABA, a neurotransmitter, decrease orgasmic ability in women, and thujone lowers GABA.

Two other innocent spices, anise and fennel, also offer sexual-enhancing qualities, but have a darker side when rendered into essential oils. Both can be narcotic and dangerous, but both also raise estrogen hormones, two obvious reasons why they earned their aphrodisiac reputation with the ancients.

Some plants' aphrodisiac reputation is more basic and nutritional. Women of menstruating age need iron for their libido. Basil, for example, is a good source of iron, especially when consumed in quantity like in pesto. Particularly if there was a shortage of red meat, basil could help make up an iron deficiency. Arugula is also a good source of iron; however, in ancient times it was the arugula seed that was used as an aphrodisiac. Arugula is in the mustard family— mustard seeds in general are high in zinc, magnesium, and arginine. Pistachio nuts are also high in zinc, magnesium, and arginine. Arginine has been shown to improve sexual function in both men and women by improving genital circulation. I've already explained the importance of zinc and magnesium.

Lizards and snails may not be for everyone's palate, but they are very good sources of omega-3 fatty acids.

The science behind carrots' aphrodisiac reputation is lost in time, because modern carrots are very different from ancient carrots. Ancient carrots were very bitter and purple, containing anthocyanin rather than the modern beta-carotene of orange, sweet carrots. Making an educated guess, I think the flavonoids in ancient carrots may have acted like some modern flavonoids, ramping up nitric oxide levels—perhaps the old purple carrot was an ancient Greek Viagra.

As for the turnip, that most prosaic of vegetables, again we have to look at the whole plant. Turnips, *Brassica rapa,* when grown for their root are called turnips. But if grown for their seeds, they are called field mustard, and it's the seeds that are aphrodisiac, for the same reason as arugula seeds.

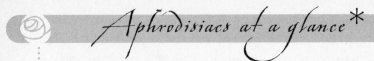
Avocado: The Aztecs called the avocado tree "Ahuacuatl," which translated means "testicle tree." The ancients thought the fruit hanging in pairs on the tree resembled the male's testicles. This is a delicious fruit with a sensuous texture. Serve it in slices with a small amount of balsamic vinegar and freshly ground pepper. The real reason it works for women: it is high in omega-3 fatty acids. It contains alpha-linoleic acid (ALA), which is a precursor to EPA and DHA. It's also high in magnesium and zinc.

Figs: The Ancient Greeks celebrated the arrival of a new crop of figs by ritual copulation. (Many believe that the shape of fresh, ripe figs resembles female genitalia: you decide.) The real reason it works as an aphrodisiac for women: it's an excellent source of iron, magnesium, and zinc. Figs were Cleopatra's favorite fruit.

Garlic: The "heat" in garlic is said to stir sexual desires. Garlic has been used for centuries to cure everything from the common cold to heart ailments. Make sure you and your partner share it together. The real reason garlic works: it triggers nitric oxide production and improves genital circulation, like Viagra.

Oysters: These tenders from the sea are often associated with Casanova but have been enjoyed for thousands of years for their apparent power to boost sexual vigor. The real reason oysters work: they are high in zinc and also, of course, high in omega-3 fatty acids, both parts of the Orgasmic Diet.

Peaches: In ancient China, the peach represented sexuality that had reached maturity and was ready to be picked. Just think of its dewy pink color, its fuzzy skin, and the juicy flesh and scent. The real reason peaches work: they are sensual to the touch, as well as high in vitamin C.

Truffles: These musty delicacies are quite expensive and are only available in season (during autumn). But they are associated with potency—especially in the groin area. Truffles smell like male pheromones. Most truffles come from western Europe and are harvested with the aid of female pigs. (Apparently it has to be female pigs, who are able to find the truffles because they detect or pick up the scent that smells like male swine sex pheromone from the truffles. Humorously enough, male swine pheromones closely resemble the male human sex pheromone; in a double-blind placebo-controlled study, women became aroused smelling it.) The real reason truffles work: they smell similar to androstenol, a sex hormone found in the saliva of male pigs (and under the arms of male humans). Again, truffles are insanely expensive. If you want to get more bang for your buck, invest in male human pheromones from the Athena Institute and spike your partner's aftershave with androstenol.

*Sources: www.GourmetSleuth.com, www.very-koi.net/food.

Changing the Way You Eat

Most of the women who are on the Orgasmic Diet enjoy it. When I've asked them if they had to radically change the way they eat, most said that they had already been adapting their diets to a more healthy one, so the foods on the Orgasmic Diet didn't seem to present too much of a challenge. And all the women were able to put their own special imprint on the diet, adapting the diet to their taste buds and choosing foods they already enjoy. One woman, Eva, from Seattle, said, "I did not have to change the way I eat all that much. I was already close to it. I still need to cut back more on carbs and eat more lean protein."

But some do come a long way. As Blaire, a thirty-nine-year-old woman from Denver, said, "I started to eat more dark chocolate but only managed to eat it around three times a week, as I don't like the taste. I started to eat much more protein and limit starchy and sugary foods. I think the only way I deviated from the diet was that

I had to continue to take birth control pills." And Roberta, a thirty-something single woman from Dallas, said, "My original dietary habits were atrocious. Fast foods, fatty convenience foods, chips, candy, caffeinated sodas. Basically I ate everything that was not good for you, and my libido was nonexistent. I changed my diet because I wanted to get healthy and lose weight. Within a few weeks of making the change, I noticed my desire for sex increased, and once I added the supplements and Kegels, it went into overdrive."

In the next chapter, you will discover what I call the orgasm killers, those foods, habits, and other factors that can get between you and your orgasm. Read on!

CHAPTER SIX

The Orgasm Killers

I know I probably shouldn't use a football analogy in a book for women, but I'm going to anyway. While fish oil may be the quarterback of my diet, the spectacular effects of fish oil are easily sacked by some modern-day libido-killers. A woman needs to be smart and avoid these offensive linemen to keep her libido and orgasmic ability in top-notch form. Here's a partial list of the main offenders: caffeine, herbal stimulants, nicotine, starchy and sugary foods, antidepressants, hormonal birth control, soy, trans fats, and omega-6 fatty acids. These are the orgasm killers, and I'm going to briefly explain their negative sexual qualities here.

Caffeine

I know what you're thinking—I can't give up *coffee!* And my recommendation isn't as drastic as all that. To give an explanation, a key part of my diet is the deliberate manipulation of neurotransmitter levels in the brain, in particular those of dopamine and serotonin. The goal is to have a high dopamine level and moderate, steady levels of serotonin. Caffeine acts on your serotonin levels like a trampoline. It causes sharp spikes of serotonin, which as you may recall, offset the sexual impact of dopamine. (See chapter 3, in which the importance of dopamine-serotonin balance is explained.) Fortunately, this spike in serotonin is short-lived and wears off in a few hours when the caffeine wears off. So you can have a lower level of serotonin at night if you only drink a small amount of coffee (one cup) in the morning. That's what I call a "workaround," and a workaround a lot of women on my diet embrace. You are in charge of manipulating your neurotransmitter levels for sexual and other purposes. You've probably been doing it instinctively all along, anyway. "I can't think of sex right now, I have to focus on the work at hand. I'm just too fuzzy. I know, I'll have a cup of coffee or a Coke!" But remember, it's that fuzzy feeling that helps with sexual pleasure. But realistically a woman can't spend her whole life in a sexual haze; sometimes a sharp focus is needed in the day-to-day world. You just need to know what you are doing on a physiological level; then you can own the process.

Some women rightfully point out that the quality dark chocolate I recommend on my diet contains caffeine. Isn't there a contradiction? It depends on how much you eat. Too much dark chocolate will act exactly like coffee and negate the libido-enhancing effects. Caffeine is caffeine. However, dark chocolate is full of all sorts of other libido-enhancing elements, so I recommend a moderate

How I Followed the Orgasmic Diet

"One of the hardest parts of the diet for me was giving up caffeine. So I experimented; when I had a lot of caffeine—like two cups of coffee in the morning and then a diet soda in the afternoon as a pick-me-up—I really could tell in the evening; I just had no libido. When I had just one cup of coffee in the morning and no caffeine the rest of the day, I still had my libido surge in the evening."

—Rita

balance, eating no more than a half-ounce of quality dark chocolate every day and keeping your coffee intake to a minimum.

Herbal Stimulants

Caffeine isn't the only thing that spikes serotonin. Other herbal stimulants do, too, like ginkgo and ginseng. I know, you are thinking, "But ginkgo and ginseng have reputations as aphrodisiacs!" Indeed they do, but in our phallocentric society, an aphrodisiac for men is considered an all-around aphrodisiac, even if works against female sexuality. Men generally do not have problems with desire. They are concerned about having rock-hard erections and having stamina in bed. Women do not care how rock hard our clitorises are and probably don't want the time to orgasm to be lengthened. High serotonin levels help with the things men need, so men may find these herbal stimulants sexually helpful. Women should avoid them. In fact, the only herbal I recommend for women for sexual purposes is the herb damiana (see chapter 2).

Smoking

Other substances spike serotonin. We are a serotonin-driven society. Smoking spikes serotonin tremendously. Now you may be saying, "But it also spikes dopamine, right? Doesn't it even out in the end?" But caffeine and smoking are similar. Both smoking and caffeine give an initial high dopamine spike that quickly wears off; then the serotonin effects are more long-lasting. Nicotine of course is also terrible for sexual function in both men and women because it constricts blood vessels. While it is true that erectile hardness is not as important to women as it is to men, still we do need good blood flow in our genital area for full sexual enjoyment. Though you can drink just one cup of coffee, very few women are able to only smoke one cigarette a day. You probably can't have just one cigarette in the morning and go cold turkey for the rest of the day, so your serotonin will ramp down by evening for a night of great sex. So yes, I am joining the loud throng who are saying, "Smoking is bad for you—cut it out!" The good news is that the high dose of fish oil I suggest may help some smokers quit, because while the oil doesn't spike serotonin levels, it does raise them to a moderate healthy level, increasing your sense of well-being and making you less reliant on cigarettes for that rush. And fish oil raises dopamine levels, too, erasing the urge for that sharp brief spike of dopamine that comes from inhaling. It's interesting to note that the smoking cessation drug Zyban is simply the serotonin- and dopamine-raising antidepressant Wellbutrin, repackaged under a different name. And although I don't have any research on a connection between fish oil and quitting smoking, we do know that fish oil acts just like Zyban does; it raises serotonin and dopamine levels. However you go about it, just quit smoking. You know you should any-how, and isn't sex more important than nicotine?

Starch and Sugar

There is also a sneaky serotonin spiker that almost every woman has to deal with—sugary and starchy food. Dr. Judith Wurtman at MIT has done extensive research on the serotonin-raising effects of carbohydrates. As I explained in the chapter on foods, meals with only carbohydrates and no fats or protein will spike a woman's serotonin levels in the same way that caffeine does. Candy and junk food will do this, but so will an entire meal of rice cakes. So eat meals with a balance of carbs, fats, and protein. Again, I am not saying you must give up all-starch meals forever. The serotonin-spiking effects of a carb-heavy meal only last for a few hours, so if you want to indulge earlier in the day you will be fine by evening. However, I should also remind you that a steady diet of all-carb meals will over time affect hormone levels. All-carb meals spike SHBG, which ties up a woman's free testosterone—see chapter 3 to refresh your knowledge of the hormone connection.

Antidepressants

The most obvious serotonin spikers are antidepressants. Except they don't just spike, they crank a woman's serotonin up to a very high level and keep it there. That's the purpose of antidepressants, and I'm certainly not saying women should go off them if they need them. It's better to have no sex drive at all than to be thinking about suicide! Particularly in cases of severe depression or depression triggered by traumatic events, antidepressants are an absolute godsend. But women often don't realize how much antidepressants can affect both their sex drive and orgasmic function. Even men, who are sexually hardier than women, are done in by antidepressants; that is, many men lose their sex drive on antidepressants, too.

In fact, antidepressants are now being prescribed to treat premature ejaculation in men because they are so effective in slowing down orgasm and reducing desire.

Finally, word is getting out about the libido-dampening effects of most antidepressants. Studies have been done showing that all of these medications have this effect, and it's no wonder, because they all have the same goal of raising serotonin levels. The one exception is Wellbutrin, an antidepressant that raises levels of both serotonin and dopamine so it does not lower libido. This makes good sense and fits in with the principles of my diet. Also, women on my diet may find that they are able to reduce and sometimes completely eliminate their antidepressant medication because of the antidepressant effect of the high-dose fish oil. Of course, do not try to go off antidepressants on your own; this should *only* be done under the supervision of your doctor. If you are on antidepressants, I strongly recommend taking the full amount of fish oil appropriate for your height and weight, and also giving the more expensive ultrarefined brands a try. I think you will be pleasantly surprised after a month or two by the beneficial effect on mood. As Kathy, a thirty-one-year-old computer programmer from New England, said, "My mood improved a lot. I feel more open, more relaxed. I used to

What Happened to Me on the Diet

"I went on the diet because I wanted a higher sex drive as well as better sexual response. When I started to feel better taking the fish oil, I consulted with my doctor and he lowered my dosage of antidepressants. He said it was fine so long as I wasn't experiencing any signs of depression or anxiety returning."

—Paige

be a hypochondriac, always worried I was about to get cancer or something. Now, after only four weeks on the diet, I am so much more relaxed and at ease with myself."

(You can check the bibliography at the back of this book for specific research studies that show how fish oil helps depression.)

Hormonal Birth Control

Much of my diet is a balancing act focusing on neurotransmitters and the various things that affect them. But hormones are important for sexual function, too. Unfortunately, hormonal birth control may have a negative sexual effect on a large number of women. Hormonal birth control contains synthetic versions of the body's natural progesterone and estrogen hormones. It works by tricking the body into thinking it's pregnant so a new egg is not released. It also thickens the cervix lining to keep sperm out and prevents fertilized eggs from implanting in the wall of the uterus. It comes in pills, patches, rings, implants, and injections, but all hormonal birth control works on the same basic principle. These synthetic hormones decrease ovary activity, including suppressing higher testosterone production from the ovaries during the middle third of the menstrual cycle. A recent study shows that not only does hormonal birth control increase SHBG, but the SHBG elevation continues after women stop hormonal birth control. Remember, SHBG binds with testosterone, lowering the free testosterone available to the body, and you want this level to remain at a healthy low.

This is a very unpopular fact, but more and more scientists are finding the courage to speak out about the negative effects of hormonal birth control on a woman's libido. Both Dr. Irwin Goldstein and Dr. Jennifer Berman have spoken out about the negative and sometimes permanent effects hormonal birth control can have for some women. (See the bibliography at the end of the book for research and studies supporting the impact of birth control on women's sexual functioning.)

Talk to your doctor about these negative sexual side effects caused by your form of hormonal birth control, and discuss the option of switching to a more low-impact type of hormonal birth control. For some women, particularly women who are not in a long-term relationship, using two barrier methods, both condoms and either a cervical cap or diaphragm, may be a better choice. I know barrier methods take away some of the spontaneity of sex, but condoms do protect against disease and you aren't going to be having spontaneous sex if you have no sex drive, anyway. Women who are in long-term monogamous relationships and who are very conscientious and methodical may find a wonderful freedom in using the sympto-thermal method (which is determined by taking your basal body temperature and tracking your cervical mucus) to determine fertile days, and using a diaphragm or cervical cap on those days. Finally, for women who are certain they are all done having children, either an IUD or a vasectomy for their partner can be the most convenient and trouble-free choice for birth control. I believe

What Happened to Me on the Diet

"At first I was reluctant to go off my hormonal birth control—I've been on it for about seven years—not just as birth control but to regulate my period. But once I started to feel such an intense sexual desire and knew the diet was working, I decided to get off the Pill. My husband and I have to be more diligent, but the trade-off is that I am thinking about sex all the time!"

—Kathy

in empowering women, and women should know that there are other forms of birth control besides the doctor-prescribed hormonal method.

Soy

Another pernicious and very common hormonal disrupter is soy. Recently, we have become a soy nation. Two sorts of people benefit from eating a lot of soy foods—menopausal women who are looking to find some relief from unpleasant symptoms and people who are embracing a celibate lifestyle. For the rest of us, soy sucks, frankly. It kills testosterone levels, and testosterone is what governs desire. Even in the case of menopausal women, I personally believe that a more sensible way to deal with the effects of dropping estrogen is to replace the estrogen with bioidentical estrogen. Bioidentical hormones are made from plants, engineered to match exactly the hormones that your body makes. I strongly recommend Suzanne Somers's book *The Sexy Years* for more information on this topic. While soy may mimic estrogen and relieve some of the symptoms caused by a drop, it doesn't affect the underlying issue—low estrogen.

Nowadays soy is in everything. Tofu and soy milk are considered health foods. Surely they are health foods—if you are a celibate Buddhist monk. Now, you don't have to avoid soy completely. A little soy here and there as an additive won't have much of an impact on your sex life. But if you are constantly eating meal replacement bars and tofu and drinking soy milk, just say no. Embrace real foods. Meat and nuts and cheese and eggs and milk are good for your body. I know it's hard with today's hectic lifestyle to always eat right, but soy is not the answer, as cheap and portable as it is. Yes, protein is important and your body needs it, but it doesn't need it in the form of soy. Dieters are hit especially hard

How I Followed the Orgasmic Diet

"I was really a soy junkie—for so long I'd been hearing about the benefits of soy for women. So when I started the diet, it took awhile to wean myself off it. But I've got to say that now I don't even miss it—in fact it feels good to be eating dairy again!"

—Blair

with soy. Many diet products, like Slim-Fast, are full of soy, because the protein it provides helps with hunger cravings. But calorie-wise, a protein is a protein. Lean red meat will work just as well and is better for you. You just have to pack your lunch instead of drinking it out of a can.

Trans Fats and Omega-6 Fatty Acids

The libido killers I just discussed—things that cause spiking serotonin and wonky hormone levels—are simply things to avoid so that you can return your body to optimal health and allow the fish oil to work. Going off caffeine, carb-heavy foods, soy, and nicotine basically helps avoid the unhealthy altered state so many women live in today. However, there is another libido killer to avoid—fats that directly interfere with the action of fish oil.

As briefly explained in the previous chapter, there are four broad different types of fats: saturated fats, monounsaturated fats, polyunsaturated fats, and trans fats. Trans fats are synthetic fats manufactured from the other fats and pose numerous health risks you. They are the fats found in junk food and commercial baked goods, and with stricter federal food labeling requirements and increased media attention of late they are being phased out of most grocery foods. Saturated fats are the sorts of fats found in meat and dairy. They have been the focus of bad publicity in recent years, but for the purposes of the Orgasmic Diet they are neutral. Monounsaturated fats are also neutral in terms of my diet. Monounsaturated fats include olive oil, canola oil, and oils from nuts. Finally, polyunsaturated fats can be divided into two groups: omega-3 fatty acids and omega-6 fatty acids. Omega-6 fatty acids are the type of fat one thinks of when hearing about polyunsaturated fats; polyunsaturated vegetable oils like corn oil, soybean oil, safflower oil, and cottonseed oil are all omega-6 fatty acids and should be avoided. Finally, of course, there are the omega-3 fatty acids found in fish oil, fish, wild game, and the omega-3 fatty acid ALA found in walnuts and flaxseed.

As you saw in chapter 3, both trans fats and omega-6 fatty acids will negate the effect of the fish oil you take. Both interfere directly with omega-3 fatty acids—but for different reasons. Trans fats are partially hydrogenated vegetable oils and are particularly bad for you, for many reasons. Omega-6 fatty acids are healthy for you, as long as they are consumed in proportion with omega-3 fatty acids, ideally in a one-to-one ratio. But the typical American diet has a twenty-to-one ratio of omega-6 fatty acids to omega-3 fatty acids.

Stress

There is another libido killer, and it's not something you eat. You can follow my diet perfectly and this will kill the whole thing (although your sex life in your dreams will be amazing!). Stress is the culprit here. I don't like to emphasize stress too much, because for the last fifty years reducing stress is the only advice women have been getting on how to improve their sex lives. I firmly believe women have been done a great disservice by the focus on this one issue, when so many, many physiological issues impact our sexuality much more—hormone levels, neurotransmitter levels, circulation, and so on. Still, just because it has been overemphasized doesn't mean stress is not an issue at all.

Stress is real and it will drop your libido, primarily because stress does impact hormonal levels and neurotransmitter levels. It's at the nexus of the mind/body connection, and actually you can use stress to monitor your orgasmic ability. Take me, for example.

I have been on my diet now for seven years and have been spontaneously orgasmic for four years. My libido is very high. My orgasmic ability is very high. Yet, because I am not in a committed relationship so soon after my divorce, I wholeheartedly embrace stress because of its libido-lowering effects. I do this to deliberately turn down my sex drive. As a single mother trying to provide for her family and also keep the house clean, the children fed, and the laundry done, I can't help but feel stress. I have a challenging full-time programming job and mountains of housework and of course I want to spend quality time with my girls in the evenings and on the weekends. Just packing lunches and making sure homework is done and pets are fed and plants watered and my car maintained and dealing with everyday household emergencies on my own without the help of another grown-up around is a daunting task. Plus, I can't be thinking about sex all the time when I have other, more pressing priorities. So not only is stress my libido-lowering friend, it's my life.

Stress is real, and it has the power to kill a woman's sex drive. A whole sex-therapy industry has been built around this one concept— the "take-a-bubble-bath" approach, as I like to call it. And for women who have their brain chemistry and hormone levels on target, the take-a-bubble-bath approach works like a charm. Whisk a woman away to a romantic bed-and-breakfast or a carefree sunny beach resort for two weeks with no cares or responsibilities and many women will find they want a lot more sex than they do at home.

More important, what many men don't seem to realize is that not only does stress decrease a woman's sex drive, but watching her husband relax while she takes on all the stressful work will also make any woman less keen to have sex. For many women, mothers especially, it is true that the best form of foreplay is to watch a man doing the dishes. The crucial thing here is that I believe women are smart. They know when they are under stress. And I strongly believe that they know when stress is negatively affecting their sex drive. Women know their bodies and they know their lives. It is insulting to tell a woman that her libido problem is all in her head or a result of her overworked lifestyle when she knows that there is something off with her body. Men aren't treated that way. When men have ED (erectile dysfunction), physical causes are the first thing investigated—not their psychological makeup.

But to truly know yourself you have to ask yourself questions. Do you wake up in the morning with a jolt and get cracking right away, only to drop exhausted into bed eighteen hours later with no respite? Is your to-do list eight pages long? My diet will help your libido whether you like it or not, but if this is how you live your life, your libido will get shoved into your dream state. Erotic dreams are nice, but actual sex is better. So, have you made a subconscious choice for whatever reason to say no to sex? Perhaps you no longer find your husband attractive, or perhaps you no longer feel sexually attractive yourself. My diet helps improve body self-image, too, but if you are living in a state of sexual denial, your subconscious can successfully repress the beneficial effects of the diet and you will just end up cranky and irritable. If you are unable to cut back your responsibilities and stress levels, perhaps due to unavoidable life circumstances, focus on getting your body into top-notch sexual form as best you can, by going on my diet. But if your situation is such

I'm not a psychotherapist, but I have consulted some professionals and gathered some commonsense ideas for how to take the stress out of our lives, sublimate our worries so they don't interfere in our ability to experience pleasure, and quite simply relax a bit so those juices can flow!

✳ **Take time to breathe.** I know, I know, this sounds like a new age cliché. But I'm talking about *remembering* to breathe. Deeply. In and out. While you're at a stoplight. While you lie in bed for fifteen more seconds before getting up to start your day. While you chop vegetables and prepare dinner. While you drive home from work in traffic. Consciously breathe in and out slowly and deeply. This has an amazing power to slow the heart rate, get more oxygen to the brain, and relax you.

✳ **Take time to exercise.** Yes, this is killing two birds with one stone: the exercise will help your libido and sexual functioning but it will also relax you, enabling you to better cope with stress. Face it: stresses don't go away; but we can learn to cope with them differently.

✳ **Take time to fantasize.** Again, you're accomplishing two things at once here. You are connecting to your inner sexual self (always a good thing in my book), and by letting your mind wander in a sexual direction, you take it away from your worries and to-do list.

✳ **Try to get the sleep you need.** Studies are showing that the body needs its sleep—to rest, rejuvenate, and replenish itself. Do you cling to those late-night hours of calm and peace? They could be working for you more if you used those hours to sleep instead of watch television, do laundry, or surf the Internet. A healthy amount of sleep is crucial to our overall health and well-being, enabling us to cope better with stress.

that you can delegate, you can find time to relax, you can say no when people ask you to take on more work, and you don't do these things—you need to ask yourself, "Why am I avoiding sex?" In this situation, sex therapy with a trained sexologist may be helpful.

I know this is a case of do as I say, not as I do. I'm deliberately choosing a stressful life. I am deliberately reducing my libido. On the other hand, I'm not currently in a long-term committed relationship, and with my very high libido and orgasmic capacity from being on my diet for so long, I have to do something to take the edge off!

A Quick Checklist for Orgasm Killers

Y N

☐ ☐ *Are you avoiding meals or snacks made of pure starch or sugar?*

☐ ☐ *Have you cut out caffeine in the form of soda, diet drinks, coffee, and tea?*

☐ ☐ *Do you check labels of processed foods to be sure they don't contain trans fats?*

☐ ☐ *Have you eliminated soy and soy products from your diet?*

☐ ☐ *Have you looked into nonhormonal forms of birth control?*

☐ ☐ *Have you implemented ways to manage the stress in your life so that it won't take over your sexual psyche?*

If you answered no to any of the above questions, then you might have to look within to see why you are sabotaging your own sex life. You know what to do!

CHAPTER SEVEN

Exercising Your Sex Muscles

As you have heard from a number of the women on the Orgasmic Diet, taking the fish oil supplements and following the Orgasmic food plan are sure ways to jump-start your libido and get you ready for fabulous sex. And many women follow the diet in just those two ways. They may eliminate caffeine or cut way back on it. They may take other supplements and indulge in their half-ounce of dark chocolate daily. But they stop there, at least for a while. And then they want more. They have begun to feel that surge of sexual power; they experience pangs of lust in the middle of the day, and they come back to me (or now, they come back to this book), looking for more—pleasure.

This is where your PC muscles come into play: If you want to fully enjoy the thrill of deep, body-shaking vaginal orgasms, ones made even more intense through the use of a simple tool that I will be telling you more about later, then you need to strengthen and tone these vital sex muscles.

What Strong PC Muscles Can Do for You

Your goal is to reach peak sexual functioning and orgasmic ability; superior PC muscle tone and genital circulation are key elements. When you tone and strengthen the PC muscles that line your pelvic floor, you will enable and/or enhance G-spot and cul-de-sac orgasms (those that you feel deep inside of your vagina), improve clitoral erectile performance without slowing down orgasm, and increase the chance of experiencing female ejaculation. One woman reported that after doing PC muscle exercises for a few weeks, she was able to experience "vaginal—both G-spot and cul-de-sac orgasms—as well as spontaneous orgasms without touching, just squeezing while thinking erotic thoughts."

But before you hit the mat and start working out your pelvic muscles, let's first make sure you are truly familiar with your PC muscles and basic Kegel exercises. Although many women are aware of their PC muscles and know the benefit of Kegels for pelvic floor health, the basics of how to tone and strengthen these "sex muscles," including where the muscles are located, what they do, and how they affect sexuality, is not always clear.

First Things First

The PC, or pubococcygeus, muscles run from the front to the back of the pelvic floor like a flat, wide rubber band. As sex educator Lou Paget suggests, a good way to locate this band of muscle is to stick your middle and index fingers into your vagina and squeeze around them as if you were trying to slow the flow of urine. Once you are able to locate these muscles, do another short exercise to get a sense of just how long they extend. The more clearly you can feel the shape of these muscles the better you will be able to access them.

1. Lie on your back with your knees bent.

2. Begin gently squeezing your PC muscles in a light pumping motion.

3. Now relax the muscles completely.

4. With your knees still bent, pull in your PC muscles in a motion from the tip of your clitoris to the back of your anus. Do this slowly and gently, not in a tugging motion.

5. The more frequently you do this, the more accurately you can feel the extent of your PC muscle band.

Benefits of strong PC muscles

Through the exercises I recommend, you will strengthen and tone your PC muscles. PC muscle strength has extensive health benefits, including:

✻ Faster recovery after childbirth due to your muscles' increased elasticity, tone, and strength. When women deliver vaginally, their PC muscles naturally stretch to accommodate the birth of the baby. If their PC muscles are already strong and toned, these muscles will return to their prepregnancy condition much more quickly.

✻ Prevention of tears or need for episiotomies after or during childbirth because of increased elasticity of your PC muscles. Again, if a woman's PC muscles are already toned and strong, her muscles can provide the stretch needed during childbirth and avoid tearing the skin.

✳ Prevention of prolapse (displacement) of pelvic organs. When the PC muscle band is stronger, it is less vulnerable to physical stress. When PC muscles become very weak and stretched too thin, pelvic organs can prolapse, causing tears, incontinence, and eventually the need for hysterectomy.

✳ Reversal or lessening of incontinence or leaking urine when you sneeze or cough. Many women, after childbirth or as a natural result of aging, experience a bit of incontinence; strengthening one's PC muscles acts as a prevention tool.

✳ Increase of the flow to the pelvic area of white blood cells, which defend the body against illness-causing viruses and bacteria. This increase in circulation in the genital area helps the body get rid of toxins and fight disease.

How to Do Your Kegels

A Kegel is a pelvic floor exercise named after Dr. Arnold H. Kegel, who in 1948 published "A Nonsurgical Method of Increasing the Tone of Sphincters and Their Supporting Structures" while at the University of Southern California Medical School. The exercise strengthens and tones the pubococcygeus muscles (PC muscles), which are attached to the pelvic bone and act like a hammock, holding in your pelvic organs. A Kegel is akin to the motion you make to stop the flow of urine.

Again, once you have located the muscles, simply tighten and relax them to get the feel of how far they extend from front to back of your pelvic floor. Then try to do the Kegel exercise.

Here's how:

1. Contract your PC muscles, squeezing them lightly for five seconds.

2. Release the muscles for five seconds. Keep in mind that it's as important to rest and relax these muscles as it is to tighten or contract them.

3. Repeat twenty-five times. If doing twenty-five repetitions
   seems too difficult, start with increments of ten.

As stated, Kegels are usually recommended as a way to strengthen
and tone your PC muscles to help with childbirth, incontinence as
women age, and overall genital health. But as you will soon see, our
main focus in this program is to use the Kegel motion with a resistance device to catapult you into Sex Goddess status! You'll soon
be able to not only achieve a vaginal orgasm, but also control when
and how you want to orgasm and even learn to have multiple
orgasms.

Becoming a Sex Goddess: Using Your GyneFlex

The benefits of strong PC muscles for overall health are clear,
and these positive effects are well within your reach with Kegels.
However, if you want to really ramp up your ability to experience

What research shows

As I and many women will attest, Kegels alone are not sufficient to build truly strong PC muscles. Studies done for urinary incontinence research, but applicable here, too, show scientific support that better results can be attained by using vaginal weight devices that provide resistance. Specifically, in a study by Drs. Jonasson Larsson and H. Pscherea of the ob-gyn department at Karolinska Insitute in Sweden, it was shown that "training with vaginal cones produced significantly better pelvic floor muscle strength than did exercise without cones." (For more complete study sources see the Bibliography.)

vaginal orgasms, learn how to orgasm when and how you want, even learn how to experience female ejaculation, then you might just want to try using a vaginal resistance device. These devices are what truly guarantee exceptional vaginal ability.

As I was researching and testing the Orgasmic Diet, I tried a variety of widely available PC muscle exercise devices for review for the Women's Sexual Health Foundation (www.twshf.com); I found the best two to be the GyneFlex device and the Kegelmaster 2000. Both are available online. My personal favorite is the GyneFlex. I find the GyneFlex more comfortable and easier to clean, but both are equally effective. Both cover about the same range of resistance—the Kegelmaster in one device, the GyneFlex in multiple copies of the same device (available in varying strengths). The cost is the same for the same range of resistance; however if you already have pretty good PC tone and can start on the medium-strength GyneFlex, you will need to buy only two of the three sets of GyneFlex, so you'll save money.

The GyneFlex is a gynecologist-designed instrument to enhance sexual arousal and sexual response, so when you combine it with the other elements of the Orgasmic Diet, you will only increase the effectiveness of the device. As Michaela said, "I was used to doing Kegels, but nothing prepared me for the impact on my orgasms once I was using the GyneFlex—I don't mean to sound like an advertisement, but that little thing is amazing! I can feel an orgasm way back inside of me—it is so intense!" And Eve, in her fifties, said, "I started with the medium-resistance #3 GyneFlex and could barely budge it. It was very difficult to get going with it but I was motivated. Now I am up to the high-resistance #5. I do twelve to fifteen minutes in the morning about five days a week. This is probably the hardest part of the program for me but I really feel it's vital."

The GyneFlex may also make having an orgasm easier, help you control the timing of the orgasm, and enable you to feel your orgasm more intensely and for a longer length of time—not bad, right? Kay, a woman in her forties, said, "I use GyneFlex for my PC muscles—now when I use it I find before long I am orgasmic and unable to concentrate on the exercise itself because I'm having several orgasms!"

By using the device regularly (twice a week for twenty minutes), you will strengthen and tone your entire pelvic floor muscles but also improve your genital blood circulation and neuromuscular sensitivity. In other words, you will feel sexual pleasure more intensely and more deeply. The more you get used to using your GyneFlex (or other resistance device), the more able (and likely) you will be to make this same motion during sex. You can massage your lover's penis and not only help to stimulate your G-spot but also to give your lover pleasure. With even more exercise, you will become more aware of any kind of genital sensation, which in turn will help you key in to your sexual sensation and translate your desire into an orgasm.

As I described above, your PC muscles extend back toward your anus, as well, and as this "hammock" of muscles strengthens and becomes more toned, you might also enjoy sexual sensation through anal sex—if this is something you enjoy. Toned muscles don't mean tight muscles. Indeed, they increase in flexibility, so anal play is more comfortable as well as more pleasurable when your PC muscles are more in shape.

Other PC Muscle Toners

Before we go on to the specifics of how to use your GyneFlex, I do want to suggest other devices that can strengthen and tone your PC muscles:

Your PC muscles will enable you to enjoy a mind-blowing vaginal orgasm even if your partner is not a man. One woman, Mandy, told me this about her experience on the Orgasmic Diet: "My partner is a woman and it was such a rush when we went on the Orgasmic Diet together. We both changed our diets, took the fish oil, and did the PC exercises with a device. We never realized that we had the power to have vaginal orgasms—it's like we had never taken advantage of all those toys we had!"

✳ Vaginal cone weights (made famous on *Oprah!*)—these are similar to tampons in shape and come in varying weights. You insert them into your vagina and walk around, clenching them to keep them in place.

✳ Kegelcisor—a stainless-steel rod that you insert into your vagina for resistance, which can be used either doing "lifts" lying down, or in a similar fashion to the vaginal cone weights, clenched while standing up (although this is an advanced technique).

✳ Kegelmaster 2000—this looks like a small curling iron that like the GyneFlex is inserted in your vagina to strengthen your PC muscles.

✳ Tantric stone egg—just like the name, this device is a smooth egg-shaped stone that can be used to strengthen your PC muscles and stimulate your G-spot; a small bit of string is attached to help pull out the device or to hang weights on for more advanced exercises.

✳ Ben wa balls—these small gold balls offer very light resistance but can be useful in developing muscle coordination once strength has been achieved with other devices.

All of these work to some degree, and they certainly can't hurt. See Resources for a complete list of stores and websites.

Using Your GyneFlex

The GyneFlex comes in three varying strengths and degrees of resistance. Elderly women or women who have recently given birth should start with the least firm White GyneFlex (levels 1 and 2 of difficulty); for most women who are sexually active, including women who have given birth in the past, try the Regular Pink (levels 3 and 4 of difficulty), and for those of you who are up to a real challenge who have mastered the lower levels, and also young women, try the most firm Blue (levels 5 and 6 of difficulty). Each color comes with two devices, in two different levels of firmness.

Before using your GyneFlex, make sure it's clean and that you are comfortable inserting it. So before beginning, you should:

1. Wash your GyneFlex with warm water and soap.

2. Rinse it thoroughly with water.

3. Dry it with a clean paper or cloth towel.

4. Coat it with Astroglide or a lubricant of your choice.

Inserting your GyneFlex is similar to inserting a diaphragm, but a lot easier since it isn't a slippery disc and the handles stay outside the vaginal opening! Here's how to insert your tiny Thighmaster:

1. First, get comfortable. Lie on your back (with or without a pillow under your buttocks, whatever is better for you) with your feet flat and your knees bent.

2. Squeeze the ribbed handles of the device together.

3. Hold the lips of your vulva apart with one hand.

4. Insert the GyneFlex into your vagina with your other hand. (The GyneFlex should be inserted so that it flexes in a front-to-back manner, not side-to-side).

Doing the GyneFlex Exericse

Essentially the motion you are doing is a Kegel, with the GyneFlex inside of you. The device adds resistance, making the Kegel more effective.

1. Just like you are performing a Kegel, squeeze the handles of the GyneFlex together. If at first nothing happens, keep trying. With practice, and as your muscles strengthen, you will begin squeezing the device.

2. Slowly and rhythmically flex the GyneFlex with a relaxation of the muscles between squeezes. If you are not able to bend the GyneFlex at all, you are using too high a level. If you are easily able to completely close the GyneFlex, you are using too low a level. Start off doing the exercises for five minutes and work your way up to twenty minutes a session.

For further information, instructions, or ordering details, contact www.gyneflex.com.

Without a doubt, using a GyneFlex or a Kegelmaster is the one step of the Orgasmic Diet that pushes women from simply accessing their libido to being able to orgasm vaginally. As Dana, a thirtysomething from Dallas, said, "I use the #3 and #4 GyneFlex regularly (twice a week for twenty minutes). I've also started using some Ben wa balls to practice gaining isolation control of my vaginal muscles. I've only been doing it for a couple of weeks. I can now have a clitoral orgasm, but these past few days, I've been beginning to feel stronger physical sensation vaginally so I'm hopeful this will lead to vaginal orgasms soon."

Another woman, Bettina, from the Boston area, said, "I've always done Kegels and I've been able to have vaginal orgasms, but nothing prepared me for how intense an orgasm could feel after using the GyneFlex. It was an entirely different feeling—just incredible! My whole body shook!"

Are you sold yet?

Female Ejaculation

Strengthening and toning your PC muscles can also lead to another strange, but quite delightful experience: female ejaculation. Less than 10 percent of women experience ejaculation, and the ability generally does require exceptional PC muscle tone. However, if you push your PC muscle development to the limit, as I have, it is very likely you too will develop this ability. The choice is yours; if the entire concept makes you feel uncomfortable, then exercise your PC muscles only moderately (don't go past the Pink level of the GyneFlex in your exercise program). PC muscles are just like any muscle—their strength and tone depends on how often you exercise. If you do find that you have the ability to ejaculate, it is easy enough to let your muscle tone lapse and lose the ability if you like. Simply stop exercising the muscles for a while, and then resume in moderation.

However, you might want to give this skill a try. Women who are able to ejaculate generally ejaculate from G-spot stimulation. The ejaculate itself is similar to prostate fluid in men and is ejaculated from the urethra. However, unlike men, women do not have a valve that shuts off their bladder, so if the bladder is full, everything comes out at the point of orgasm—urine along with ejaculate. I advise women who can ejaculate to empty their bladders before sex.

Female ejaculation feels, at least initially, a lot like you are losing control of your bladder. There is a lot of mental resistance and early conditioning to be overcome in having your first ejaculation. Some women find themselves thinking back to their early years of being potty trained and how they learned to "hold it in." I often recommend that women first get comfortable with the idea that what is in your bladder will come out the first couple of times. You can practice by yourself in bed (put a thick towel down) or in the bathtub—having a glass of wine or beer may help you relax both physically and mentally. Then stimulate yourself with a device that accesses your G-spot such as a thin glass, steel, or acrylic dildo made for G-spot stimulation, typically curved, and often called a wand. A fast tapping motion is generally best, with a thin, hard toy. The orgasm feels dirty, but good. Once you know what ejaculating feels like, you can do it with an empty bladder so only ejaculate comes out.

All Exercise Enhances Sexual Pleasure

When you get your blood flowing in any way—whether by walking briskly through your neighborhood, taking some deep breaths, running a mile or two, or taking a yoga class, you naturally help your sexual vigor. Any kind of physical exercise increases stamina and improves circulation of blood through your body; this automatically will have a positive impact on your sexual responsiveness.

Why exercise?

* An increase in stamina and energy will help you make sexual interludes last longer.

* Sex will be more playful and fun because your endorphins are increased.

* Improved flexibility will enable you to be more inventive and creative with sexual positions.

✳ You will be able to hold positions for longer lengths of time, enabling you to give more pleasure to your partner.

Exercise also helps us relax, counteracts stress, and improves our overall well-being—all of which help us get in the mood and stay in the mood for sex. As an aside, because women do need moderate and healthy levels of serotonin to avoid depression, one of the best ways to achieve steady serotonin levels is simple physical exercise. While a woman may need to do more strenuous exercise to build muscle tone and lose weight, for the purposes of healthy brain chemistry a simple stroll will do wonders, especially if it is outside in the sunshine. The key is to walk for at least a half hour at a time. I mention this only in passing. My diet has plenty of steps; daily walks are not part of the official program.

But it is true that moderate daily aerobic exercise worked as well as an antidepressant in raising serotonin levels in mildly depressed women (see page 186 in the Bibliography). In addition to making it easier for women to cut back on unhealthy serotonin spikers, moderate aerobic exercise also has the added sexual benefit of improving circulation, and while improving genital blood circulation isn't the be-all and end-all for women like it is with men, it certainly can't hurt! The more blood we have flowing down there, the more feeling we are going to experience.

Moderate aerobic exercise also raises dopamine levels, particularly low-stress exercise like a leisurely stroll or yoga. So regular moderate exercise is a good thing all around for sexual purposes. "Beginning to exercise, even walking forty minutes three times a week, makes me feel better," reports Carla, age thirty-five, married and the mother of three. "I've never liked to work out, but I do enjoy being outdoors. Also, the exercise seems to fit with my new way of eating. But the best part is how much more energy I have and more in touch with my body I feel—it all makes me feel more sexual, more attractive."

Personally I like both yoga and, although I feel goofy doing it, the aerobic video game Dance, Dance Revolution. Both can be done at home when convenient, both get blood flowing and raise dopamine levels, and both improve body awareness.

It's clear both from my anecdotal research and other investigation that women with strong PC muscles do show a higher percentage of vaginal orgasm ability. However, strong muscles all on their own won't necessarily bring vaginal orgasm ability; a woman has to be able to feel the improved sensations from stronger muscles and increased blood flow, which is why strengthening your PC muscles is just one part or step of the Orgasmic Diet. In order for you to feel a sexual sensation from your strong and toned PC muscles, you need to have proper dopamine-serotonin balance, which as you know by now, comes from eating right, taking fish oil supplements, *and* exercising. It is a whole body program—and the results will change your *whole* life.

a truly satisfying sex life

PART THREE

CHAPTER EIGHT

Getting in Synch with the New You

The Orgasmic Diet has changed my life. Over the past seven years, I have been transformed from a self-conscious, insecure, dependent woman into a self-assured, confident, passionate dynamo. Please excuse me if I sound boastful. It's not that I think I'm the grandest dame around, but rather that I want you to feel this way, too—and you can.

If you've reached this point in the book, and you've been following my plan, then you are probably undergoing your own transformation. For some women, the transformation is loud and big and you want to shout from the rooftops (I think I fall into this camp); for others, the changes are more subtle, taking place in their minds as well as their bodies. These women look more directly at themselves when gazing in the mirror; they answer questions with more clarity and affirmation; they walk more resolutely down the street. And they have more fun, passion, and pleasure when having sex. So many women have shared that since being on my diet, they just feel different, and this difference makes them feel so good. But with those good feelings come other changes, changes that need to be integrated into our selves, our lives, and our relationships.

More Energy

Our sexuality is a core part of who we are as women, as humans, and as individuals, so it is natural that as this part of us changes, we will feel different in our skin. As Kris says quite simply, "My self-esteem has gone up. I think it's due to the fact that I've lost so much fat and am feeling more lively. I don't feel as lethargic throughout the day as I used to."

Like Kris, many women feel more physically fit and vital on the diet. Although those women who do lose weight have been thrilled by this added bonus, the physical impact of the diet is not just a weight issue. It's an all-over energetic issue. Women, myself included, simply have more energy to do things when they are on the plan; they are more focused and clearheaded; and they get more done. This is great because it creates more time for having sex, right?

So when you begin to notice that you feel better and have more energy, make a conscious decision to save some of this energy for sex. I know this is tired cliché, but if you don't plan on sex, it just doesn't happen—especially when we all live such busy lives with so many competing commitments.

Mental Adjustments

Some women have shared with me mixed feelings about the changes they've been experiencing since starting the diet. Though by and large they welcome their new sexual vitality and power, some have had to let go of parts of themselves that no longer really fit. As Eve, a woman in her early fifties, shared with me, "I've had to make some mental adjustments. I've lost some things but gained a lot. Even though the new stuff has been a lot of fun it took a while to accept the loss of the old ways. My husband and I have discovered some new sexual positions that we both like *much* better than the straight missionary of the previous thirty years. I'm much more focused on intercourse now than I was, though foreplay is still great, too."

Here, Eve is referring to having to let go of the sexual comfort zone she had had with her husband. With her stronger libido and recharged sexual responsiveness, the long hours of cuddling with her husband don't happen as frequently; they are fornicating like bunnies instead! Just kidding—well, almost. Like many women, especially those old enough to have established entrenched patterns in either their relationships or in the way they think about themselves, moving out of their comfort zone takes some adjusting—like rearranging the furniture in your brain.

One woman shared with me that it was actually difficult to get used to feeling so self-confident. "It was as if I kept looking for that shadow self to reassert herself and say, 'You're not the real Louann. You're an imposter.' I knew this was my old voice just wanting me to second-guess myself. I guess sometimes I still can't believe I really can do all of this—can have so much pleasure from sex—after so many years of feeling absolutely nothing."

My advice is to give yourself some space and some time to adjust to this new you. Don't expect to be transformed mentally right away, and don't be too hard on yourself if you don't get the effects you hope for. Be kind to yourself and just let things happen.

The Diet and Your Relationship

All of these changes will necessarily and inevitably impact your relationships. Almost every woman with whom I've spoken, been in touch with via the Internet, or met personally has said that without a doubt, regarding the results, her partner has been "ecstatic," "elated," "all for it!," "psyched about it," and even a subdued, "very pleased." Another woman, whose partner is a woman, said this, "We've been together for almost ten years, and sexually things between us were getting kind of boring. We were drifting apart and we knew our intimate relationship needed a real boost. The Orgasmic Diet was just what we were looking for—but now our friends never see us because all we want to do is stay home!"

Basically, the partners of these women are eternally grateful and enthusiastic supporters of the rich sexual transformations that their women have undergone through the Orgasmic Diet.

But again, change is change, and I believe it's always best to be prepared for change rather than freak out when changes happen. So here's some advice.

Sharing the News

Some women went on the diet without telling their partners. Some of these women did so because they were afraid to get their partner's hopes up if the diet didn't work. Others were unaccustomed to talking about sex in their relationship, so as a matter of course, they did not "share" the news that they were trying to rekindle desire. And still others simply wanted to keep the information private until they were ready to share. As Rita, a fortysomething woman from Washington, said, "I had not told him that I was on the diet at first. But he definitely noticed a change and was very pleased—and quite amused when I finally told him." Kathy, a thirtysomething woman from New England, said in almost a confessional tone, "I was afraid to tell my husband at first. I didn't want him to get his hopes up. He was trying to be supportive and understanding but I just knew that he was really frustrated that I never wanted to have sex. Now that I'm on the diet, he's so much less moody and more patient—we've both changed!" In general, I always think it's best to be totally up front, particularly when it comes to sex. Sex is after all an intimate act—intimate physically, emotionally, psychologically, and for some, spiritually. But of course, the decision is up to you.

How You Feel

Many women who begin the diet because they have no libido and great difficulty reaching orgasm also feel extremely dejected. They may have little or no self-confidence. They have lost touch with themselves. They might even feel unhinged in their lives in general. If you're in this emotional situation, you might also feel alienated from your partner or husband—who wouldn't? Of course, I know this situation intimately. My lack of sexual power had eroded my self-esteem and self-worth and I had determined (quite unconsciously at first) that I was of less value than my husband because of this. It makes total sense that in this situation women might feel quite desperate about their relationships. As one woman confided in me, "I had tried everything and nothing worked and I was really scared that my relationship was just going to fail because of *my* low libido and lack of interest in sex." All of this can lead to fears or feelings of alienation from your partner.

You need to know two things if you are in this or a similar situation. First, you are valuable, you do have power, and you will see—by virtue of this diet—that you will be in control of your sexuality before long. You will not only become reacquainted with your libido but you will feel more sexually alert and desirous. You will feel this, not just think this. And the longer you are familiar with these feelings and sensations, the more able you will be to believe in your new power. As you grow in self-confidence, you will also gain (or gain back) your sense of power in your relationship. It may not have gone anywhere; you might just have thought it disappeared. Regardless, you will have a new sense of equality in your relationship.

Second, if you are in a truly loving relationship, then your partner will want you to be a sexy, sexually empowered woman. He will cheer your newfound desire and get on his bended knees to give you the thrill of an orgasm!

The two—sexual empowerment and your partner's enthusiasm—will more than likely go hand in hand.

Show Him You Care

I know this sounds obvious, but while on this diet, on any diet for that matter, it's easy to get so focused on you and the changes within your body that you might lose sight of your other half. If you tell him how the diet is impacting you, you will not only turn him on, you might blow him away! He can't guess at your desires; you have to make sure he knows what they are.

Suggest Something New

Once you have confidence and your partner's attention, you might also want to suggest something new: a position, a toy, an erotic movie for foreplay. In other words, take advantage of your new energy and enthusiasm and be creative. You will quite possibly find yourself more curious and more confident to test new waters of pleasure.

Treat Your Relationship as Special

God knows relationships require work. But the sexual dimension of your relationship can be a place where the two of you can retreat to relax, grow more intimate, and have some fun, too! This requires a conscious decision and commitment. We are all very busy. We always have "more important" things to do than focus on our relationship. Every time you push away the opportunity to have sex with your partner, you push away the chance to be close and reenergize your relationship. Sex is powerful. It creates tremendous energy that can heal, cement, and deepen relationships. Make sex a part of your daily lives.

If the Problem Is More Personal

"But wait," you might be saying to yourself, "I went deep into myself and found out the real reason my libido is gone is my husband/boyfriend. What do I do now? A diet's not going to help that!"

You'd be surprised. In some ways women are not all that different from men. When a guy is sixteen, pretty much any woman with a pulse looks attractive. Just saying the word *boobs* can give a sixteen-year-old guy an erection. Old, young, pretty, ugly, thin, fat—when a man is sixteen, if a woman of pretty much any description wants to have sex with him, sex is going to certainly going to cross his mind in a very vivid way. As men get older and their libido and orgasmic capacity decline, they get more particular. By the time they reach a certain age, many men find that only women who fit their ideal can get their blood stirring. And of course deep love also helps.

This is very politically incorrect of me to say, but women also have this sliding scale. We just don't hit the top of it very often, while men generally do as a matter of course while going through puberty. If you don't find your partner attractive anymore, ask yourself if you find any men attractive. A woman with a high libido who is no longer attracted to her partner will find other men sexually appealing. Not that she will necessarily act on her desires, but she will definitely notice men's sex appeal.

If you no longer find your partner attractive and you have stopped noticing other men, too, you need to ask yourself the uncomfortable question—are you subtly or subconsciously sabotaging your libido through physical and mental means? Some women are subconsciously fearful of straying in a marriage or relationship and will instinctively choose lifestyle and dietary choices that effectively shut down their libido. They may also put up a mental fence around sex and arousal. This generally backfires, because most men are not going to be happy with a woman who has lost all desire for sex with them, even if she is completely faithful.

I don't have answers for how to navigate this situation. Sometimes perhaps the choice of asexuality is the best for some women and some relationships. I certainly believe that if a woman feels her husband isn't romantic enough or physically attractive enough or dominant enough or muscular enough or even simply "new" enough, she will be surprised at how her standards change as her libido climbs. Suddenly the same old husband can become very sexually attractive indeed and all of those missing elements are forgotten. But with a climbing libido may also come the awareness of the attractiveness of other men. I firmly believe that in the end love conquers all, and women will be most attracted to the man they love the most if the love is strong. I also believe that an increasing libido can be a tremendous catalyst for change for a woman who might be trapped in a bad relationship, a bad marriage. If it's a lack of respect from your man rather than his lack of biceps that is causing your drop in libido, finding your own sexual power is a strong force for freedom and coming to your own determination of what's best for you.

I'm not saying that you are wrong if you feel deep down it's a lack in your partner that's causing your drop in libido. It's an uncontestable truth that a hottie-hot hottie is going to make even the coldest woman's heart jump up and take notice. Whether that hottie is your husband or partner or not is a question only you can answer. But reawakening your sexual fire may help you figure out what you truly want. In any case, listen to what your subconscious and your body are telling you.

By and large, women on the Orgasmic Diet feel empowered, more centered, and more able to cope with their lives in general. As Paige, age thirty-seven, said, "I discovered that sex can be great and that my body is capable of so much more than I previously thought. The sex was way better for me." That's it in a nutshell!

For me, going into a sexual encounter with absolutely no doubt in my mind that I will easily orgasm has transformed sex. There is no performance anxiety; I can concentrate on pleasure and fun. And my desire is so high I have great freedom in choosing whom to be with; it doesn't have to be Mr. Absolutely Perfectly Right. He can be Mr. Right Now. In my daily life I have confidence and a Mona Lisa smile on my face, knowing how powerful I am inside.

CHAPTER NINE

Clitoral Orgasms 101

So far, the main focus of my diet has been to show you how to increase your chances for experiencing a vaginal orgasm. Indeed, I am very enthusiastic about your learning this skill, and I strongly encourage women to strive to master it. However, the gold standard for women's orgasms is the clitoral orgasm. This is what most women learn first, and what they rely on for pleasure. Of course, my diet helps you with both types of orgasm, but in different ways. But even after increasing their genital circulation and enhancing their PC muscle strength and tone—two positive side effects of my diet—some women still have trouble experiencing a clitoral orgasm. So to that end, I have added this bonus chapter in hopes of helping you increase your pleasure during a clitoral orgasm.

Many women are capable of having clitoral orgasms, even if they have female sexual dysfunction (FSD), and only a small percentage of women physically can't experience a clitoral orgasm as a result of surgery or nerve damage from trauma to the region. Others are unable to have clitoral orgasms due to genetics and natural development of the genitals; but again, both conditions are quite rare.

Yet even women with a good, healthy libido may have difficulty having clitoral orgasms. As some women hit perimenopause or menopause they suddenly develop difficulty in having clitoral orgasms; these women mourn this sudden loss of pleasure and are dying to find a way to resensitize their clitoral area. And for the woman who has never had an orgasm of any kind, the quest for a clitoral orgasm is usually first on her "Want One" list, which is why the clitoral orgasm deserves special attention.

So whether you have never had a clitoral orgasm, have them but only with great difficulty, or used to have them and want them back, this chapter is for you. For those of you who enjoy clitoral orgasms, you still might want to take a glance at this chapter—it is chock-full of helpful information that may enable you to prolong, deepen, or widen your clitoral orgasm.

If You've Never Had a Clitoral Orgasm

There are a number of reasons some women never have a clitoral orgasm. The primary one is lack of practice. If you feel strong sexual desire, if you get aroused from kissing and foreplay, if you have no problem with vaginal lubrication but you've never had an actual orgasm, generally this can be overcome with technique and practice.

The easiest way to have a clitoral orgasm during sex is to already have identified what one feels like and the particular stimulation that does it for you from masturbation practice. Therefore, an easy fix is to simply masturbate.

There are lots of books on self-stimulation methods, but I think the practical and direct approach is the best. If you've never had a clitoral orgasm, simply buy a vibrator, a very strong vibrator, and use it on yourself. I recommend the Eroscillator. Although it is very expensive (about $100), it is incredibly stimulating and one of the most powerful vibrators you can buy. It's also almost completely silent, never overheats, is submersible, comes with a variety of quality silicone attachments, and makes a handy dildo if you remove the attachments.

If the Eroscillator is too pricey for you, the Hitachi Magic Wand is also excellent. If price is really an issue, a cheap bullet vibrator may do the trick for under $15. In any case, simply hold the device against your clitoris and an orgasm should soon be forthcoming, after a few sessions of practice, or perhaps even immediately. But in my experience communicating with hundreds of women, the Eroscillator is particularly effective for women who have never had a clitoral orgasm.

I recommend initially using your vibrator regularly, at least twice a week. This will give you experience in exactly what a clitoral orgasm feels like, which in turn will make it easier for you to reach orgasm from manual stimulation. Spend several months regularly reaching orgasm with a vibrator, so your body gets used to orgasm and comes to expect it or need it. Often, once women get familiar with having orgasms, their bodies want them all the time.

If you are in a sexual relationship, after the first month of achieving regular orgasms on your own you can incorporate your vibrator into sex, if you and your partner both feel comfortable with that. You may find that you can more easily have an orgasm with the vibrator when you are alone than with a partner—indeed, some women are unable to have a clitoral orgasm in front of their partners. This is perfectly normal, especially for women who are new to orgasm.

Some women feel embarrassed or ashamed at the thought of masturbation. I say that what's good for the gander is good for the goose. Virtually every man prepared his body for sexual intercourse by years of masturbation, by learning his sexual response and orgasmic triggers through practice. Knowing they can reach orgasm is a big part of what gives men sexual confidence in the bedroom. Women can have this same confidence by learning to have a clitoral orgasm on their own. Once you know you can orgasm solo, you know you can orgasm with your partner during sex. Think of it like playing scales so you can play the piano: the more you practice, the less nervous you will be on recital night.

If you are still feeling uncomfortable about masturbating or about relaxing enough to reach an orgasm with the stimulation of a vibrator, then you might need work with a sexologist to overcome psychological blocks to self-pleasure. It also may be helpful to read pro-masturbation books, such as Betty Dodson's *Sex for One,* Barbara Keesling's *Sexual Pleasure,* and Lou Paget's *The Big O* (see Resources for a full listing of titles).

When Clitoral Orgasms Are Hard for You

For many women, it's still very hard, though not impossible, to have a clitoral orgasm, even with a very skilled and patient partner focusing on clitoral stimulation. The difficulty stems from a variety of causes, often working together. Consider the possibility that you may have one or more of these physiological conditions.

Lack of Blood Flow to the Clitoris

Poor genital blood flow will inhibit your ability to have a clitoral orgasm or needlessly limit the intensity of your pleasure while having one. Going on my diet will improve circulation, which is particularly important with clitoral orgasm difficulties. Exercising the PC muscles will also improve blood flow in your genital area. The clitoris itself is not just an external nerve structure. The clitoris actually extends back six inches into the pelvis. I like to explain to men that giving women a clitoral orgasm is analogous to trying to give themselves an orgasm while only being allowed to touch the head and frenulum of their penis. The majority of our clitoris nerve endings are buried deep in our body, only able to be indirectly stimulated through the vaginal walls, so when blood flow is increased, your nerve endings are more easily stimulated.

Weak PC Muscles

If your PC muscles are weak from lack of use, then this might also be contributing to lack of sensation in the clitoris. Strengthening the PC muscles through Kegels or with a GyneFlex-like device allows a woman to directly stimulate the rest of her clitoral nerve structure by flexing the muscles below the clitoris during stimulation. Strong PC muscles may serve to delay orgasm, but will also increase the strength of the clitoral orgasm and build arousal.

Dehydration and Low Blood Pressure

I don't have direct evidence for this, but after years of listening to women describing their sexual difficulties and asking for sexual advice, I strongly suspect that low blood pressure and dehydration play a part for many women who have difficulty with clitoral orgasms. A good number of women with low blood pressure who have a high libido and are easily aroused but have great difficulty reaching clitoral orgasm have told me that after drinking rehydration drinks, they experience improved clitoral orgasm. So although my evidence is purely anecdotal, there seems to be a connection. If you know you have low blood pressure and it's okay with your doctor, then try to drink more fluids (water!) throughout the day and raise your electrolytes (sodium, potassium, chloride, and bicarbonate).

You may want to try rehydration or sports drinks, which contain not only necessary fluid but also electrolytes. I prefer unflavored Pedialyte over Gatorade because of the lower sugar content. Even if you can't stand the taste of these drinks, try drinking at least eight ounces a day for a couple weeks. If you notice improved clitoral responsiveness, you will see the hydration factor at work.

Desensitization

If your clitoris has lost sensation due to age or decreasing hormone levels, or both, you may respond very well to a resensitization aid. Many women have tried Viagra, and it does work for some, although it failed clinical trials on women. You can ask your doctor for Viagra, but my anecdotal research suggests that Viagra simply increases blood flow to the clitoris without increasing sensation, and actually may delay orgasm—not a good thing for us. Luckily, there are also many topical creams that help with resensitization. I have tried many of them myself out of curiosity, and the most effective and the only one that I know of that has passed clinical trials is a topical herbal oil called Zestra, but you should see what works for you. A few drops of this oil applied to the clitoris will most definitely increase clitoral sensation and responsiveness, without slowing down orgasm. It smells nice, too, although strong—a pungent, deep floral scent.

If your clitoris has lost sensation due to trauma or surgery, Zestra may also be helpful, particularly if the trauma or surgery has restricted blood flow to the area.

However, the most common reason for desensitization is easily remedied. Simply stimulating the clitoris too intensely and too frequently can cause desensitization and an inability to reach orgasm from oral or manual stimulation during sex. The most common culprit—vibrator overuse. Fortunately this is easily overcome through a practical approach listed below, starting at step 2.

One type of masturbation-induced desensitization some women have is caused by a particular masturbation style, involving riding a pillow or the corner of the bed to reach orgasm. This type of masturbation style makes it very difficult to reach orgasm from oral sex or manual stimulation, but on the other hand it lends itself well to the sex act itself, if the woman can grind in a similar manner on her partner's pubic bone during sex. Many women with this type of desensitization are content with the fact that intercourse is better.

Go for It: Learning How to Have a Clitoral Orgasm

Once you have more insight into the physical reasons that may be causing your difficulty having a clitoral orgasm, and you've addressed the issues under your control, then you are ready to really learn how to have a mind-blowing clitoral orgasm. Go for it, but remember, practice makes perfect. So in order to get you up and running, I have outlined a kind of miniprogram. I tackle the purely physical aspects first, then the practical, and then the psychological, from easiest to hardest.

Mastering the Clitoral Orgasm

1. If you are new to orgasms, you need to keep experimenting until you find the best way to bring yourself to orgasm alone; initially, the easiest and most fail-safe way is with a very strong vibrator.

2. After several months of having regular orgasms with a vibrator, it's time to decrease the intensity. Lower the speed of your vibrator. You may now find it easier to reach orgasm if you cut back the frequency of vibrator use so as not to desensitize your clitoris.

3. While you work to master clitoral orgasms from lighter stimulation, you should also work on your powers of erotic concentration and fantasy. Read women-oriented erotica to give you ideas and put you in a sexual mind-set. Erotica and porn are actually very helpful in getting you into a sexual frame of mind and giving you material for your imagination. *The Red Shoe Diaries* and other soft-core porn films are recommended. You might also want to sample Candida Royalle's Femme line of erotic films made especially with women in mind. *Playgirl* also produces some sexy films. In terms of written erotica, there are many excellent sources, including Violet Blue's Best of series, as well as her book, *The Smart Girl's Guide to Porn.* Good online sources of erotica include The Erotica Readers & Writers Association at www.erotica-readers.com, Clean Sheets at www.cleansheets.com, and *Libido* magazine at www.libidomag.com.

4. After you hone your erotic concentration and stimulate your clitoris through lighter and lighter vibrator touch, it will be time to switch to your hand. By the time you come to the point of transitioning from a vibrator to manual stimulation, you should have an idea of how often your body is able to orgasm. A good rule of thumb is that a woman in her twenties can climax as often as every day to twice a week; a typical woman in her forties achieves orgasm three times a week to twice a month (though going on my diet may push you toward the more frequent range). These ballpark numbers are for solo orgasms; orgasms during sex are generally half as frequent. These ranges are very rough; there is a huge variation between women's orgasmic rates. The important thing is to find your body's natural rate. If when using a vibrator you generally want and have an orgasm every day, that's your orgasm rate. To successfully resensitize your clitoris, you have to drop down to one-seventh your orgasm rate. I call this the resensitization frequency. So, for example, if you are having an orgasm every day with your vibrator, to resensitize you have to temporarily cut back to only having an orgasm once a week—then you will be more likely to achieve clitoral orgasm with your partner and no vibrator, though more on that later.

5. Now you're ready to box up your vibrator and put it in the closet. Every day practice your erotic fantasizing; read erotica to get you in the mood or, even better, have sex with your partner to really get you in the mood. Then take time for yourself, but no more than twenty minutes of manual stimulation of your clitoris. Generally a fast flicking motion, done lightly and steadily, is the most effective. As Barbara Keesling recommends in her book *Sexual Pleasure,* speeding up your breathing rate and gyrating your pelvis can also add to your arousal level. If you still are unable to orgasm, get yourself as close as you can and finish with the vibrator on its lowest setting. Make sure that if you need the vibrator to climax, you are only having orgasms at your resensitization frequency. In other words, if you were regularly having

orgasms three times a week with your vibrator, drop back to having an orgasm only once every two weeks. This is very hard to do and requires willpower, particularly when you are deliberately arousing yourself with fantasy, but the result is worth the wait. Eventually with enough practice and enough orgasmic steam built up, you will always be able to have an orgasm without your vibrator.

6. Once you have made the transition from orgasming with a vibrator to orgasming with your fingers, gradually increase your orgasmic frequency until you are at your normal masturbation (with a vibrator) orgasm rate. In other words, if you had to cut back to once every two weeks to reach your resensitization frequency, see if you can increase the rate of your orgasms back to your previous orgasm rate of three times a week. Spend several months at this level until your body gets used to it. Don't use your vibrator at all—keep it boxed up in your closet.

When a woman learns how to have an orgasm as easily with her fingers as with a vibrator, she not only betters her chances that she can be stimulated by her partner—manually, orally, or through coital alignment technique (see page 149 for details on CAT), but she also increases her sexual confidence. Being able to self-stimulate means you know your body. It means you know how you like to be touched. This self-knowledge is empowering and vital for full sexual satisfaction.

Get Creative

Once you have mastered the art of self-stimulation, you are now ready to take your clitoral orgasms to a whole new level.

1. Start varying your masturbation stroke, making it lighter, less steady, less focused on the clitoris only.

2. Spend time touching other parts of your vulva and other parts of your body.

3. Slow down your stroke and keep honing your erotic fantasy focus. See how long you can prolong your masturbation session without losing erotic focus, and see how aroused you can get before you even touch yourself.

4. Change the position of your body. If you always have an orgasm flat on your back, try having an orgasm on your side, or lying on your belly or sitting in a chair. Try to have one standing up, which can be very difficult but is certainly worth a try. Trust me.

5. During this process it is also helpful to cut back your masturbation rate, not drastically, but maybe in half. Gradually increase the frequency until you are able to have an orgasm with a completely different stroke and body position each time. You may find your natural orgasm rate with these new methods is somewhat lower than your orgasm rate back when you were using a high-powered vibrator to orgasm, but you can now climax in lots of different ways—a true bonus!

Adding a Partner to the Mix

Whatever your new rate, once you have spent several months with this wide variety of stimulation, you are ready for the biggest leap—having an orgasm in front of someone else. You may feel uncomfortable with this interim step of self-pleasuring in front of someone else, but it is a helpful step on the path to resensitization. It allows a woman to get over the feeling of performance anxiety with a sexual touch she is already confident about. Women associate self-pleasure with something they need to keep private and hidden, vestiges of another era when women were taught to hide their sexuality. Now I know none of those outdated ideas are impeding my readers, right? Think of it this way: most men (and women, too) find watching their lover pleasure herself an extreme turn-on. With these simple steps, you'll be closer to becoming orgasmic from the stimulation of your partner's hands and mouth.

Each of the following steps follows the same general formula as for self-pleasure. First find your natural rhythm. Then, cut back to your resensitization frequency so that you build up orgasmic steam, one-seventh your normal rate. Then over a period of weeks try new methods. As your body becomes more comfortable orgasming in the new way, gradually increase the frequency back up to your regular orgasm rate with the new technique. Once you feel comfortable orgasming at your normal rate with the new technique, you can move on to the next step. It is a very time-consuming process and can take a long time, but the rewards are worth it.

1. Focus on mutual masturbation—have your lover stroke himself while you break out that vibrator that has been collecting dust boxed up in your closet. The first few times you do this with your partner, a glass of wine may bring comfort. Perhaps watch an erotic movie to get the focus off you. After a long period of lighter self-stimulation, the more intense stimulation from the vibrator should help you lose any performance anxiety.

2. Now it's your partner's turn to use the vibrator on you. And remember, allow your partner to pleasure you—keep your hands to yourself, and close your eyes and fantasize.

3. Once you feel comfortable with your partner holding a strong vibrator and giving you an orgasm, move to a lighter vibrator or dial down the intensity of the vibrator you are using.

4. Next try manual stimulation, but go back to mutual masturbation.

5. When you feel comfortable manually stimulating yourself to orgasm in front of him, have your lover manually stimulate you, showing him, in a loving, patient way, exactly how you stimulate yourself.

6. Keep up this process, forcing your body to move to a higher level of sexual response before you reach orgasm. And experiment with a variety of types of manual and oral stimulation, in a wide variety of positions.

7. Enjoy your newfound confidence!

After so much work achieving clitoral orgasms, sex becomes easy and fun! This process does require a tremendous amount of patience and trust. Associate the pleasures of orgasm with your partner. This surrender of autonomy and power can help to make your orgasms even easier—but only do this if you feel mentally comfortable. Recent research using brain scans at the point of orgasm show that female orgasms require activation of a part of the brain associated with trust—men's orgasms do not.

Of course, the steps I recommend here are rather involved and they take time; if you find your body is responding more quickly, you can speed up the process and skip steps. Listen to your body and use common sense. Your instincts won't steer you wrong.

Overusing Your Vibrator

Although I'm not saying that you have to give up vibrators for the rest of your life once you can easily orgasm without them (alas, that wouldn't be much fun), you do need to be careful as to how and when you use them. Every so often it's fun to have multiple orgasms, seven or even fifteen in a row, with the kind of electric and shocking orgasmic intensity that only a vibrator can deliver. But if you indulge this way often enough that orgasms during sex fly out the window, you may be forcing a switch you aren't willing to make. So use your own judgment and pay attention to your body.

Overuse of a vibrator can lead to desensitization. So if you begin to indulge yourself a bit too often, you may unwittingly be making it more difficult for your clitoris to respond to sensation, especially from manual or oral touch.

The vexing thing is that most women don't realize that frequent masturbation with a vibrator can desensitize their clitoris. Many think that it is becoming harder to have an orgasm because something is psychologically wrong. This is not the case. Rather, the problem is caused by too-frequent masturbation with a vibrator. When women have this problem, they find sex arousing, but with clitoral desensitization they are unable to find release. Over time, sex with high arousal without ever having an orgasm will make a woman incredibly and deeply frustrated. If the resensitization process I recommend doesn't do the trick, a vibrator can be used during sex. If you get to this point, use the vibrator for sex, and not alone.

Clitoral Orgasms During Intercourse

Just about every woman, whether it is easy or hard for her to have a clitoral orgasm from manual or oral sex, will find it impossible to have a clitoral orgasm from intercourse unless there is also clitoral stimulation happening at the same time. Men should realize this and accept it. It's just basic female anatomy; the clitoris is located too far away from the vaginal opening. But of course, having simultaneous orgasms during sex is a fun thing to do—as long as you don't feel pressure and turn this into a stress-causing issue, then give it a try. It is a fun goal. Here are the four ways for a woman to have a clitoral orgasm during penetration.

1. Have your partner stimulate your clitoris during sex while you are on top.

2. Try one of those tiny silicone vibrators attached to elastic straps that allows hands-free stimulation of your clitoris while allowing full access to your vagina. Alternately, you can try an Eggstasy Pouch, which holds a small "bullet" vibrator in the same position. (A bullet vibrator is just like it sounds, a small vibrator in the shape of a bullet or a small tampon.)

3. Stimulate your clitoris yourself during sex. Some women have an aversion to doing this, but if you don't, it is the easiest and most obvious way to have mutual orgasms. An entire book has been

Coital alignment Technique

This description of the coital alignment technique is based on the one found in Barbara Keesling's book *Sexual Pleasure*.

1. Lie on your back and have your partner lie on top of you, entering you in the missionary style.

2. Next, have your partner place his hands on your shoulders and move his entire body up toward your head about two inches. This position will enable your partner's penis to press onto your clitoris.

3. Staying locked in this position, have your partner begin to move, thrusting up and down in your vagina rather than in and out.

4. This thrusting motion will enable your partner to bring himself to climax while your clitoris is being continually stimulated. Some women reach a delightful clitoral orgasm this way!

written about this one concept, *Five Minutes to Orgasm Every Time You Make Love*, by Claire Hutchins.

4. Finally, try the coital alignment technique (CAT). This is the hottest of all the approaches, as the man is quite literally giving you an orgasm by the motions of his body, as the base of his penis rubs against your clitoris. However, it is quite tricky and takes practice (see the boxed text on the previous page).

Women who have no trouble attaining clitoral orgasms are probably rolling their eyes if they have even made it this far into the chapter. Yes, some women do have this much difficulty letting go, trusting, and simply taking the steps to learn how to have a clitoral orgasm. Most women can learn; it just takes practice!

CHAPTER TEN

A Quick Recap

As I've mentioned throughout the book, you can do the Orgasmic Diet in any way you wish. Women tend to do the diet in three phases, starting with the fish oil and other supplements. Taking a supplement is fairly straightforward, does not require much planning, and doesn't challenge you to change your lifestyle very much. In general, most of the women I have been in contact with have told me that they began to see results (i.e., their libidos were awakened and invigorated) in two to three weeks. Once they get a taste of an enhanced or newly active libido, they are encouraged to take the Orgasmic Diet a step further; this is when many women begin thinking about cutting down on starchy carbs, increasing their protein, cutting out caffeine and other stimulants that interfere with their sexual functioning, and adding their daily half-ounce of dark chocolate.

When women pair the fish oil with the Orgasmic Diet food plan, they tend to feel clearer and more energetic, and increasingly their minds turn to sex. This awareness, along with more sensitivity in the clitoris and vagina, usually spurs the final phase or step: exercising the PC muscles using a resistance device such as the GyneFlex. When women bring those PC muscles into shape, whammo! They're in for a whole new world!

So are you ready to begin the Orgasmic Diet? What follows is a quick recap of how most people follow the program. Again, you can always adjust the diet in any way that feels comfortable.

1. First, fish oil. If you do nothing else, take the fish oil and a multivitamin. It's important to take a multivitamin along with the fish oil to get antioxidants, because of the potential for fish oil to oxidize. I know I recommend a lot of pills; for the typical woman, six pills a day, and for larger women, up to eleven. Start off with the multivitamin and just one fish oil pill a day for a week. The second week, increase to two fish oil pills, and so on. Remember, it's best to take your supplements with food. If you have trouble swallowing pills, you can get fish oil in liquid form to take with a spoon.

Some women are extremely motivated and embrace the whole diet and exercise right from the start. If you fall into that camp, that's great. But for women who want to ease into the program, just taking the fish oil is a good start.

2. I see the next logical step in the program being to cut out most of the soy in your diet—no tofu or soy milk; no soy-enriched snack or energy bars; no veggie burgers that are made up of soy.

3. The next step I recommend is also relatively easy, although it does mean more pills. This is to get the RDA of calcium,

magnesium, and zinc, which usually means taking three more pills. These are easy to find; all drugstores carry them. Try to take them at a different time from your multivitamin, though you will continue to take the multivitamin, too. I generally recommend women take the multivitamin at breakfast with a third of their fish oil pills, a calcium/magnesium/zinc pill and a third of the fish oil pills at lunch, and two calcium/magnesium/zinc pills at dinner with the rest of the fish oil pills. You do need your calcium anyhow, you know you do. This is just another reason to take it. Make sure your multivitamin also has the RDA of vitamin D, to help with the absorption of all of these minerals.

4. Next, add half an ounce of quality dark chocolate daily. This isn't usually a hardship; quite the contrary, in fact. One woman on the diet says she likes to think of her chocolate as just another supplement. When I asked her if that was because she didn't like the taste of the chocolate, she said, "On the contrary, I like it too much. I take my supplements after breakfast, once I'm at work. If I had a whole chocolate bar to contend with, I don't know if I'd have the willpower to resist. This way, I break off my two squares of dark chocolate and put it in a Baggie with the rest of my day's supply of supplements."

5. Now, I encourage you to pay close attention to your body and your libido. Any sparks flying? Pangs deep in the caverns? You are probably beginning to feel a return of desire, or you are beginning to set the stage for its return. If you take this next step, I promise you will feel your libido surge like a tidal wave within you: cut down on starchy and sugary foods and cut out the caffeine. Don't just take my word for the antisexual effects of caffeine and sugary and/or starchy meals. Pay attention when you drink coffee and when you don't, pay attention to how you feel sexually after you eat a meal of meat and nonstarchy vegetables as opposed to pasta with pastry for

dessert. Pay attention to what your body is telling you! Judge for yourself. That way you will have the motivation (or not) to follow the Orgasmic food plan. If you notice that your libido drops significantly after a starchy meal or five cups of coffee, then you will know for yourself.

6. Watch your iron intake. Although iron is a minor part of the diet, most women who menstruate don't get enough iron in their diet, and low iron can have a serious impact on female sexuality. Listen to your body. If you are still menstruating, try taking a low dose of extra iron every few days for a month. See if it improves your libido and orgasmic function. If it does, continue. (Of course, women who have hemochromatosis should never take iron supplements). Check with your doctor to find out if you have this condition.

7. Exercise, exercise. That really is the sticking point for many women. And you don't need to do the vaginal exercises if you don't want to! I'd say that over half the women who go on my diet don't. If you are only interested in increasing libido, then there is no harm in skipping them. But I really do encourage you to try them. It's only twenty minutes twice a week, and you can read or watch TV while you do them. If you get the vaginal cone weights you can even do housework while you do them, if finding time is an issue.

Doing the PC toning exercises will increase your vaginal sensation during sex, make you tighter, and make your clitoral orgasms stronger and easier, and if you stick with it, may give you the ability to have vaginal orgasms, too. What you do is up to you, but for optimum benefit, exercise is key.

8. The next step is usually the most controversial part of my diet: consulting with your physician or health-care provider about whether or not you can change your antidepressant medication

and birth control method. As I mention in the chapter on fish oil, you may find that taking a high dose of fish oil will enable you to decrease and even perhaps stop taking antidepressants, under your doctor's supervision. If you are taking hormonal birth control strictly for birth control purposes, you may want to consider other options (see chapter 6), but again, only do so under your doctor's supervision. Even if you choose to stay on or are advised to stay on antidepressants or hormonal birth control, you may be surprised to see how well the diet will work in spite of these handicaps. Give the diet a chance, even if you just follow part of the plan.

9. And, finally, if you are smoking—QUIT! I know it's hard, but really, at least cut down for general health reasons. I know I'm making fish oil sound like a cure-all, but you may find it easier to cut back while taking fish oil because of your improved dopamine and serotonin levels.

Generally women do find the pill-taking part of the diet the easiest to stick to, probably because it's also the most effective. The common mistake women make on the diet is to get hung up on the foods and caffeine. Starchy carbs and sugary foods do lessen libido, just as caffeine does. But really the core components of my diet are the fish oil (and multivitamin) and the calcium/magnesium/zinc. So concentrate on the pill-taking first; it's the easiest and most effective part.

If you follow the diet, you will more than likely feel positive results in both your libido and your sexual responsiveness fairly soon (within two to three weeks). However, if you follow the diet for more than a month and you don't experience any significant positive change in your sexuality, then you may need to consult your doctor to have your hormone levels checked, specifically your testosterone (see chapter 11 for further information about hormone replacement therapy). In most cases, my diet does increase free testosterone so that both your libido and sexual responsiveness will be increased, but in some cases, women need extra help.

Ways Out of Your Hormonal Soup

While the Orgasmic Diet does work for many women, it does not work for all women. And the main reason is because the low levels (for various reasons) in their bodies of testosterone cannot be repaired by my diet.

Typically a woman's problem with testosterone has more to do with her level of free testosterone, and it's the free testosterone that affects libido. Free testosterone is the testosterone left to circulate after most of the total testosterone has been bound up with sex-hormone-binding globulin (SHBG). My diet does help increase free testosterone. It lowers SHBG, which frees up more of the total testosterone. The three things that help lower SHBG are the zinc in the calcium/magnesium/zinc, avoiding starchy and sugary foods in the diet, and avoiding hormonal birth control.

However, the Orgasmic Diet does seem to help with total testosterone, too. There is some preliminary research that shows fish oil improves testosterone levels, as does eating the healthy fats recommended on my diet. Still, total testosterone levels is the weakest link of this diet, and some women may need to take some extra measures. If you think that's the case with you, then read on.

Testosterone: The Weak Link

I strongly believe that for some women, bioidentical testosterone replacement therapy (TRT) is necessary to reach full sexual potential. Some women are just naturally low in total testosterone, some women diminish their total testosterone through diet or lifestyle, and some women lose their total testosterone due to menopause or adrenal problems or from having their ovaries removed during a hysterectomy (the adrenal glands and ovaries produce testosterone in women).

Childbirth, particularly if you give birth more than once, can also permanently diminish total testosterone levels. Remember, testosterone governs libido.

Testing and Finding the Right Doctor

The best way to determine if one's testosterone levels are low is to see an endocrinologist, gynecologist, or other doctor who specializes in women's hormonal issues. Although bloodwork will show total and free testosterone, the levels of testosterone should also be assessed within the context of a full background on a woman's sexual response, interest, and so on.

The trick is to find the proper doctor. Intrinsa failed clinical trials, so the only testosterone treatments available right now are FDA-approved treatments for men. Treating women with testosterone is off-label, not approved by the FDA. Therefore not every doctor is willing to prescribe it. I recommend the website www.fsdinfo.org, particularly the message board for references to suitable doctors in your area. Specifically, you are looking for testosterone-friendly doctors who know their way around a hormonal blood test.

On the FSD website, you will find a wealth of information on research done on testosterone supplementation in women, opinions of various doctors on this treatment, women's stories, and detailed information on understanding lab results. Also you will find recommendations for good books about treating sexual dysfunction and relationship issues. A few books that deal specifically and in depth with off-label testosterone treatment of women are *For Women Only: A Revolutionary Guide to Overcoming Sexual Dysfunction and Reclaiming Your Sex Life,* by Jennifer and Laura Berman; *The Hormone of Desire: The Truth About Testosterone, Sexuality, and Menopause* by Susan Rako; and *I'm Not in the Mood: What Every Woman Should Know about Improving Her Libido,* by Judith Reichman.

It is key to point out that the tests for women's testosterone are based on tests used with men. The results don't transfer very well, as our levels are so much lower. So for women it is very important to have the most accurate bloodwork possible when measuring testosterone. The equilibrium dialysis method is preferred for women testing their testosterone levels. If your doctor does not have a lab using the equilibrium dialysis method for testosterone measurements, you can suggest Quest Diagnostics. Quest uses an even more sensitive test, using chromatography/mass spectroscopy, the gold standard.

For any testing you might have, it is important to get the normal ranges from the lab to see where your results fall on the spectrum. Some recommended hormonal tests are:

✳ Total and free T by equilibrium dialysis (EqD) if possible—to test total and free testosterone.

✳ Thyroid function tests (TSH, thyroxine/T4)—to test function of your thyroid; some thyroid dysfunction impacts libido.

✳ Prolactin/PRL—a blood test that measures the amount of the hormone prolactin.

✳ LH/ICSH—this test evaluates your body's production of LH (luteinizing hormone).

✳ Estradiol—this test measures one of the estrogens, estradiol.

✳ FSH (follicle-stimulating hormone)—this hormone is an estradiol precursor.

✳ SHBG (sex-hormone-binding-globulin)—this test is obviously crucial to your sexual functioning.

✳ DHEAS—hormone that is a precursor for testosterone and estrogen, and also androstenedione.

If, together with your physician, you have decided that TRT is right for you, then you need to know that bioidentical testosterone (bioidenticals are hormones that exactly mimic the body's own) comes in a wide variety of forms—in pills, patches, creams, lotions, and sublingual drops (drops you put under your tongue). From what I have heard, delivery through the skin via a patch, cream, and drops works better than taking a pill. If your doctor determines that you need more hormones than just testosterone—if he or she also wants you to get estradiol, for example—he or she may direct you to a compounding pharmacy (a pharmacy that makes prescriptions on-site following your doctor's prescription, instead of using already-synthesized mixtures or blends) that can make the correct mixture for you.

The process of finding the right doctor and the right compounding pharmacy can be a daunting shopping expedition. If you need testosterone, it is very much worth it, since women who have low testosterone who start in on supplementation report not just improved sexual function, but more energy and confidence and enjoyment of life.

Testosterone Replacement Therapy— Is it Safe?

Recently a bioidentical testosterone patch for women, called Intrinsa, failed clinical trials. Although it did show a mild statistically significant improvement in libido over placebo, there was concern over the health effects of long-term male hormone replacement therapy (HRT) in women, due no doubt to the fear caused by the long-term research on more typical HRT of female hormones at menopause. I use the terms "male" and "female" hormones loosely, because of course women's bodies make testosterone, just as men's bodies make estrogen.

However, I think it's important to point out that the negative health effects from long-term HRT have only been seen in patented pharmaceuticals and not in bioidentical HRT. When looking at the long-term use of bioidentical estrogen and progesterone replacement therapy, only beneficial health effects have been seen. Suzanne Somers has written two informative bestselling books on the topic of bioidentical hormone replacement therapy, *The Sexy Years: Discover the Hormone Connection: The Secret to Fabulous Sex, Great Health, and Vitality, for Women and Men,* and *Ageless.* In *The Sexy*

Years she points out the great good sense of taking hormones that exactly mimic the body's own, rather than something like Premarin derived from horse urine—non-bioidentical hormones simply treat the symptoms of menopause and other disorders rather than giving the body what it needs—true hormones. Somers also recommends cycling the hormones to mimic the menstrual cycle.

I think it was unfair for bioidentical TRT to be judged by the long-term effects of non-bioidentical estrogen and progesterone therapy. Of course, caution in health matters is laudable, but this reluctance to approve bioidentical treatments like Intrinsa to me sounds more like a moral decision by the government rather than a genuine health concern (particularly when considering the panoply of obvious negative effects from taking Viagra). Bioidentical hormones are chemically the same as hormones produced by the human body. I do think monitoring should be done to keep the bioidentical testosterone within normal female levels, and many doctors agree that the health benefits of bioidentical testosterone treatment in women with low total testosterone far outweigh any theoretical and unproven risk.

While there isn't a set level of free testosterone that is optimal for all women, measuring your levels can at least let you know if you are on the right track. There is one negative health effect from bioidentical testosterone treatment that does make sense. The problem with taking testosterone, whether it's bioidentical or not, over long periods of time is that it causes the body to stop making its own testosterone. Bodybuilders and sports figures have been pushing the envelope on steroid use, sometimes much too far, and it's wise to learn from them. For women with almost nonexistent testosterone, there is no harm done in taking TRT under a doctor's supervision because there is no naturally generated testosterone to worry about losing. This in particular applies to women who have had their ovaries removed or have gone through menopause—you don't have to worry about losing something you don't have.

But women who have somewhat normal testosterone levels but decide, with their doctor, that TRT is right for them to ramp up their libidos should consider cycling their TRT. Follow the lead of body-builders who take testosterone vacations and use methods to kick-start their body's own testosterone production during treatment breaks. As I said above, I believe cycling HRT is a good thing in general and should also be followed when taking female hormones, so you can give your body a break just as it has in its natural menstrual cycle.

Take a look at the big picture. Did you have a sudden drop in libido after a hysterectomy? Was there a sudden drop in libido after menopause, or after giving birth? Now nearly every woman has a drop in libido at these times. In particular, the breast-feeding hormones absolutely kill a woman's sex drive. But do you still feel like avoiding sex six months after your baby has weaned? Or maybe you haven't experienced a drop in libido because you have never had a libido, and you simply can't understand what all the fuss over sex is about. All of these situations are pretty good indications that TRT should be considered. Just be smart about how you pursue this kind of treatment.

Back to the Orgasmic Diet

Another reason TRT doesn't always work is that the body tries to compensate. As total testosterone goes up with the outside supplementation, the body often simultaneously raises SHBG, making the TRT a wash. Your total testosterone may shoot up to the maximum healthy level, but your free testosterone might stay low and unbudging, so there will be no increase in desire for you. What to do?

That's where my diet comes in. The Orgasmic Diet works very well in tandem with TRT because it keeps SHBG low. And of course it enhances all the other physical issues that come into play as it increases your sexual response.

Testosterone is not a cure-all, and in fact it is so tough to isolate who it works for, and why, that scientists generally have had great difficulty *proving* that TRT works, because for many women it doesn't. But for the women for whom it works, it really, really works. So trust yourself and take responsibility for exploring the possibilities—listen to what your body is telling you.

CHAPTER TWELVE

FAQs

Q: What does a vaginal orgasm feel like?

A: In the same way a clitoral orgasm feels somewhat like a sneeze, a very good sneeze, a vaginal orgasm feels like a full body shiver, a very good full body shiver. The two main areas that trigger vaginal orgasms are the G-spot, a couple of inches in on the front wall of the vagina, and the cul-de-sac, the semicircle up above the cervix. Sometimes women who have their G-spot stimulated ejaculate during orgasms, especially if they have very strong PC muscle tone. Ejaculation orgasms feel quite strange, especially at first, but very pleasurable.

Q: I've never experienced an orgasm during intercourse; will the Orgasmic Diet help me do that?

A: The Orgasmic Diet helps women acquire vaginal orgasmic ability and improve existing vaginal orgasmic ability. After you have achieved the necessary PC muscle tone through exercise, the rest of the diet should help trigger the process leading to vaginal orgasms. Once you are able to have spontaneous vaginal orgasms from flexing your PC muscles, you may even achieve vaginal orgasms while both you and your partner remain still.

Q: Will the Orgasmic Diet improve my ability to have a clitoral orgasm?

A: The Orgasmic Diet improves clitoral orgasmic ability in three ways. First, it greatly increases libido, which makes clitoral orgasms easier to achieve through the sheer force of desire. Second, the fish oil I recommend improves blood flow to the genital area, increasing the sensitivity and ease of stimulation to the clitoral area. And finally, the PC muscle exercises in this program greatly improve blood flow to the area, which can also enhance a woman's clitoral orgasmic ability.

Q: I am never able to stick to a weight-loss diet; why should I be hopeful that I can stick to this diet?

A: The Orgasmic Diet is easy. It contains many of the foods you are probably already eating and enjoying. At first, you may have trouble reducing or eliminating caffeine, but remember you can have one cup in the morning without interfering with a plan to have sex that evening. The key is to eat balanced meals: have protein at every meal, cut down on nonvegetable carbs. It is best to limit carbs in general; simply avoiding lots of starchy and sugary foods for four or five hours before sex will still have a positive impact on libido and sexual response. This approach will not yield the optimum low SHBG levels, but it will keep serotonin levels low for better sexual activity.

Remember, the Orgasmic Diet is not a weight-loss diet. You are free to eat as much or as little as you are comfortable with.

Q: Will I lose or gain weight?

A: That depends on how you follow the program, and how much this eating pattern is an improvement on your old way of eating. But it's safe to say that most women who are on the diet have either maintained their weight or lost weight.

Q: What about my relationship—will my husband like this diet?

A: That all depends on your husband or partner, but generally men are delighted with the results. Some men are surprised at how effective the diet is and find they want to go on the diet, too!

Q: Can I adapt the diet to my liking?

A: Of course—you have total control over how much of the diet you want to follow. If you want to start out slowly to get a mild sense of how the diet impacts your libido and sexual response, then by all means start slowly. If you want to experience a strong effect, do the full program. You can always cut back on the amounts of supplements you take and modify the diet to tailor your sexual response.

Q: Isn't it bad to eat too much chocolate?

A: It is actually bad for the diet itself to eat too much chocolate, because chocolate contains caffeine. That's why I limit women to a half-ounce a day. Of course you can eat more if you desire, just watch your own body's reaction.

Q: Is it okay to have some coffee?

A: Many women go on the diet and continue to drink coffee. The diet will help even if you do continue to drink coffee, just not as much. Often women who go on the diet and drink coffee find that they start to wake up more to erotic dreams, sometimes orgasmic dreams. Once the coffee wears off during the night it frees up a woman's body to feel the full effect.

Simply, you should not drink coffee for six hours before you plan on having sex.

Q: What about diet soda?

A: Diet soda has not been seen to raise serotonin levels like sugar does. In this case, caffeine-free diet sodas would have no impact on the diet or its positive effects on your sexual functioning. However, you still need to avoid caffeinated diet drinks—the same rules apply as for coffee.

Q: I don't want to give up my vibrator; can I still use it to pleasure myself?

A: Giving up a vibrator isn't part of my diet, it's just something I've found over the years is helpful for those women who have difficulty having an orgasm during sex from manual or oral stimulation. A woman who has no problem having an orgasm from a short amount of oral sex will have no ill effects from using a vibrator as often as she likes. However, many women find that overuse of vibrators does increase the amount of stimulation required to reach orgasm during sex without one. If you are one of those women, I do recommend a period of abstinence from your vibrator; slowly add it back into the mix once full sensitivity is regained, and using it sparingly as a fun extra, not a sexual staple.

Q: How long will it take for me to feel the effects of the diet?

A: For some women it can take up to four weeks, but a great many women have felt changes in ten days to two weeks.

Q: You suggest that your diet helps to stabilize mood. I am on antidepressants for anxiety. Is it safe for me to go off them if I go on the Orgasmic Diet?

A: Only go off antidepressants gradually and under your doctor's supervision. And try a month at the full dose of fish oil before attempting to wean yourself off antidepressants.

Q: Can I take Requip or other dopamine-increasing drugs instead of fish oil?

A: I am extremely reluctant to recommend drugs like this. In the case of women who are on high doses of antidepressants and find that fish oil does *not* help them to reduce their need for antidepressants, then Requip or bromocriptine might be helpful in addition to fish oil, if closely supervised by a doctor. But for a woman not on antidepressants, I think fish oil is the safe and healthy choice.

Q: Is it okay to take so much fish oil if pregnant or nursing?

A: Check with your doctor. I believe it's actually important to take fish oil during pregnancy—DHA in particular helps with fetal brain development. However, you must be absolutely sure that the product you choose is the purest and most refined possible, to remove all the contaminants found in fish (which is why pregnant women are advised not to eat fish, because of the mercury content, etc., from our polluted oceans). In the case of pregnant or nursing women, I would only recommend the specific brands Omega-Rx fish oil from Zone Labs, or Minami.

Q: Are omega-3 fatty acids the reason for the fish oil? I ask because I can't take fish oil; it makes me break out terribly regardless of brand. I do take a tablespoon a day of flax oil,

which has comparable amounts of the same fatty acids—will
that work?

A: Flax has ALA, which is a precursor for EPA and DHA. But you need to ingest thirty times the amount of ALA to get the same amount of EPA and DHA found in fish oil, so no, the ALA in flax can't replace it.

Q: Is it possible to get the same results from the GyneFlex if you don't "hold" each rep? I've been holding for twenty seconds each rep, but it would be sooo much better not to have to count "one Mississippi, two Mississippi" and so on, and just distract myself with TV instead!

A: You can get comparable tone just from flexing; you don't have to hold. I recommend a rhythmic flexing for twenty minutes.

Q: Why is soy protein not advised for this diet?

A: Soy protein is very bad for the libido. It alters hormone levels.

Q: I have a Kegelmaster. Would that suffice or is there something about the GyneFlex that produces better results? Would using it every day be too much?

A: You can use the Kegelmaster every day if you like; but like any muscle group, your PC muscles will strengthen faster if you take at least a day off between workouts to allow for muscle growth. The Kegelmaster 2000 is equivalent to the GyneFlex; I just find the GyneFlex more comfortable and easier to clean.

Q: How much fish oil should I take if I want to start slowly?

A: I recommend a range of fish oil depending on weight—from approximately 1700–3400 mg EPA and 1300–2600 mg DHA. I'm tall and overweight so I take high end—if you are short and thin, try for the lower end. Start by taking one capsule a day with food, adding a capsule a week until you are up to the full dose for your weight and height.

Q: I want to know if using topical progesterone will counteract your nutritional recommendations and diet. I am forty-eight, premenopausal, and use Kenogen, a topical progesterone oil that works wonders for me.

A: I am against hormonal birth control when there is nonhormonal birth control—cervical cap, diaphragm, IUD, even the sympto-thermal method—that doesn't disrupt a woman's hormonal balance. But hormonal treatment for a medical condition is a different issue. Unless you noticed a steep drop in libido when you went on Kenogen, indicating that it's somehow interfering with your testosterone, it seems fine.

Q: I would love to try this diet but I'm a vegetarian and do not consume animal products. Does flaxseed oil or some other source of omega-3 fatty acid have a similar effect?

A: The best vegan fish oil is Omega Zen, but it only contains DHA and not EPA. It should still give good benefits, though it tends to be pricier than non-vegan.

Taking It All the Way

I started this book with a personal account of my sexual experiences before I discovered my diet. In describing the plan and the benefits, I have tried to pass on information I have learned over the years from other women. Since I discovered the diet I have kept my ear to the ground and studied the most effective practices, the best products, how women really feel about sex and their partners, and the many sexual difficulties they face. I have passed on what I learned to a whole new group of women with this book.

Now I'd like to share the second half of my own personal testimonial. I feel a bit uncomfortable doing so, both because I am not writing under a pen name and also because my story sounds rather outlandish. However, I am sharing my experience here in case other women experience similar effects after being on my diet for many years and because I want to show what's truly possible. I should also say I've taken my diet to the extreme, to the point of outright goofiness. I am at the highest safe maximum dose of fish oil for my weight and have extremely strong PC muscles, and of course, I follow the rest of my diet. I'm not sure why I take it so far, maybe because for so many years I couldn't orgasm at all during sex. So now, I'm comically horny and ridiculously orgasmic. I honestly have forty or fifty vaginal orgasms a day, which *is* downright silly . . . but fun. I can orgasm from just flexing my PC muscles for ten seconds or so and fantasizing—it's like a magic trick. I've even gotten good at faking not having an orgasm. I've found having an orgasm whiles away the time waiting in line or during boring meetings. And commuting to work is never dull! Of course, an orgasm doesn't happen spontaneously; I do have to be thinking sexual thoughts and I do have to flex my muscles. But with my sky-high libido, sexual thoughts are never far away. I also am amused by how my libido makes just about all men appealing in one way or another. I am continually smitten by the inherent deliciousness of them all. It's cheerful and naughty to be this way, and also gives me an incredible sense of inner power and confidence.

When I have sex with a man I orgasm instantly upon penetration, with no foreplay, and I keep going from there, every twenty seconds or so. Indefinitely. And thanks to my ability to orgasm just from flexing, I orgasm during foreplay, too, from kissing on down. Men do seem to focus on this ability of mine. It's been hard for me to find the right fit. I do best with men who practice tantra; their openness about powerful female sexuality is helpful, and of course their stamina is a plus. Ahem.

A lot of times when I talk about my abilities, women are taken aback. They think forty orgasms a day must mean I have time for nothing else. But when you can have ten orgasms in five minutes or have hands-free orgasms as easily as breathing during boring parts of your day, it doesn't seem so odd. My clitoral orgasm rate is normal, two or three a week. It's of course much easier having clitoral orgasms now than it used to be for me, thanks to my diet, but the frequency is well within the typical range for a forty-year-old woman.

I also have developed ejaculation ability. This took some getting used to, but I must say it's extremely naughty-feeling and fun and makes me feel a certain camaraderie with men (particularly because I always want to roll over and go to sleep after having one). The most peculiar thing that's happened to me sexually is that I've had a sort of tantric awakening. I am certainly not qualified to teach anything about tantra; if you are interested in learning about it I highly recommend Margo Anand's books, particularly *Sexual Ecstasy* (see Resources) and www.tantra.com. I've spoken with some tantrikas who tell me I am doing it all wrong, that orgasms must be conserved to preserve sexual energy. I can't help feeling the opposite, that the large number of vaginal orgasms I have somehow generates sexual energy. It feels as if I can create a ball of energy at the base of my spine, and then visualize it moving up my spine to various parts of my body, including the top of my head. I can release this energy at various points along the way, and this release of energy feels peculiarly like an orgasm, just an orgasm centered someplace else besides my vulva. These points correspond to the points on the body called chakras in tantric tradition. In particular I get intense sexual enjoyment from releasing this energy from the center of my chest.

Other women on the Orgasmic Diet have reported similar feelings of awakened sexual energy and chakra sensations. The tantric practitioners I've discussed my diet with have told me that this sort of energy awakening, known as kundalini rising, should only be done under a tantric teacher's guidance, and it can lead to emotional trauma if not done correctly. Personally I feel it is a very natural and basic feminine process, that our bodies know how to handle it, but I thought I should mention their warnings here.

Because I am so easily orgasmic and easily aroused, it's sometimes very confusing. If I am attracted to man I can have an orgasm from a hug, a handshake, even simple eye contact. Before I went on my diet there were only two men who were ever able to give me an orgasm; I was open to sex for the most part, but physically didn't feel much. Now I can have more sexual pleasure from brief eye contact than I used to have from hours of skilled and hot sex. This does blur the lines between what is and isn't sex, but in a fun way that takes flirting to a new level.

My abilities and libido also give me a certain feeling of power in the bedroom. I know without a doubt that I will always have great orgasmic sex no matter whom I'm with. I can relax and have fun and focus on what pleases me, without having to worry about my body being able to keep focused or stay aroused. There is a sexual equality in my actions now that I really enjoy. Some men find this intimidating, some men find it disturbing, and some men find it amazingly erotic. It's hard to predict the reaction I'll get, even if the man knows all about my abilities beforehand. A lot of men do like feeling that they are in control of giving the woman her orgasm. That's not the case with me, as it is all too clear that I'm the one in charge of my orgasms. So on the one hand I am sexually independent; on the other hand I am unbelievably and single-mindedly phallocentric. Male anatomy now gives me such incredible and intense pleasure that I simply love being with men. Men seem to find my burning attention surprisingly gratifying. I think on the whole my duality balances out—I may not be under a man's sexual thrall when it comes to orgasm control, but a lover can bring me to my knees just by unzipping his pants.

My strong muscles and enhanced sensation also have made worries about fit a thing of the past. While of course the tight entrance to my vagina is irretrievably gone after two births, farther inside I am able to grip tightly or open up to fit. And I can have orgasms from my G-spot, only a couple inches in, or my cul-de-sac, all the way at the top of my vagina. I'm adaptable.

One of the most profound changes sexually has been that I've lost that little voice in my head asking, "Am I aroused enough? Will I have an orgasm? Is he worried I won't have an orgasm? Did I turn off the oven? Do I have to set the alarm to get up tomorrow?" or saying, "God, look at my cellulite!" That's all completely gone. Now it's just, "Wow, he's hot. And he obviously thinks I am. Look at that cock! Mmm. That's going inside me right now. Oh, oh OH!" I love being this way. It's silly and fun and easy and deep and really, really hot. Join me. Let the Orgasmic Diet do for you what it has done for me. You won't be sorry. Good luck and great orgasms!

Resources

Websites

Sexologists
www.sexologist.org

Testosterone-Friendly Doctors
www.fsdinfo.org
www.twshf.org

General Female Sexuality Reference
www.bermansexualhealth.com
www.twshf.com

Tantra and Developing Strong PC Muscles
www.tantra.com

Fish Oil
www.minami.com
www.zonelabsinc.com
www.gnc.com

Omega-3 Fatty Acids

www.eatwild.com
www.oilofpisces.com

PC Muscle Exerciser and Toys

www.gyneflex.com
www.kegelmaster2000.com
www.babeland.com
www.goodvibes.com
www.evesgarden.com
www.eroscillator.com
www.womynsware.com
www.mykm.com
www.bettydodson.com

Relaxation Music

www.brainsync.com

Female-Friendly Erotica

www.a-womans-touch.com
www.erotica-readers.com
www.cleansheets.com
www.libidomag.com

Other Products

www.zestraforwomen.com
www.athenainstitute.com

Aphrodisiac Trivia

www.gourmetsleuth.com

Books

Allende, Isabel. *Aphrodite: A Memoir of the Senses*. New York: HarperCollins, 1998.

Anand, Margo. *The Art of Sexual Ecstasy: The Path of Sacred Sexuality for Western Lovers*. New York: Tarcher Putnam, 1989.

————. *The Art of Sexual Magic: Cultivating Sexual Energy to Transform Your Life*. New York: Tarcher Penguin, 1996.

————. *Sexual Ecstasy: The Art of Orgasm*. New York: Tarcher Penguin, 2000.

Berman, Jennifer, and Laura Berman. *For Women Only: A Revolutionary Guide to Reclaiming Your Sex Life*. New York: Henry Holt, 2001.

Blue, Violet. The *Smart Girl's Guide to Porn*. San Francisco: Cleis, 2006.

Bright, Susie. *The Best American Erotica 2006*. New York: Touchstone, 2006.

Colbert, Stephen. *Alpha Squad 7: Lady Nocturne*. New York: Toby & Sons, 2007.

Dodson, Betty. *Sex For One*. New York: Three Rivers Press, 1996.

Goldstein, Andrew, and Marianne Brandon. *Reclaiming Desire: 4 Keys to Finding Your Lost Libido*. Emmaus, Pa.: Rodale, 2004.

Keesling, Barbara. *Sexual Pleasure: Reaching New Heights of Sexual Arousal and Intimacy*. Alameda, Calif.: Hunter House, 2005.

————. *Sexual Healing: The Complete Guide to Overcoming Common Sexual Problems*. Alameda, Calif.: Hunter House, 2006.

Ladas, Alice Kahn, Beverly Whipple, and John D. Perry. *The G Spot and Other Recent Discoveries About Human Sexuality*. New York. Holt, Rinehart and Winston, 1982.

Leiblum, Sandra R., and Judith Sachs. *Getting the Sex You Want: A Woman's Guide to Becoming Proud, Passionate, and Pleased in Bed*. New York: Crown, 2002.

Love, Patricia, and Jo Robinson. *Hot Monogamy: Essential Steps to More Passionate, Intimate Lovemaking*. New York, Penguin Putnam, 1994.

Mohanraj, Mary Anne. *Aqua Erotica: 18 Stories for a Steamy Bath*. New York: Three Rivers Press, 2000.

Muir, Charles, and Caroline Muir. *Tantra: The Art of Conscious Loving*. San Francisco: Mercury House, 1989.

Murnighan, Jack, Genevieve Field and Rufus Griscan. *Full Frontal Fiction. The Best of Nerve.com*. New York: Three Rivers Press, 2000.

Paget, Lou. *How to Be a Great Lover*. New York: Broadway, 1999.

————. *How to Give Her Absolute Pleasure*. New York: Broadway, 2000.

————. *The Big O.* New York: Broadway, 2001.

————. *The Great Lover Playbook.* New York, Gotham, 2003.

————. *Hot Mamas.* New York: Gotham, 2004.

Rako, Susan. *The Hormone of Desire: The Truth About Testosterone, Sexuality, and Menopause.* New York: Three Rivers Press, 1996.

Reichman, Judith. *I'm Not in the Mood: What Every Woman Should Know About Improving Her Libido.* New York: William Morrow, 1998.

Schnarch, David. *Passionate Marriage: Keeping Love and Intimacy Alive in Committed Relationships.* New York: W.W. Norton, 1997.

Schnarch, David, and James Maddock. *Resurrecting Sex: Solving Sexual Problems and Revolutionizing Your Relationship.* New York: HarperCollins, 2002.

Sears, Barry. *Omega Rx Zone: The Miracle of the New High-Dose Fish Oil.* New York: ReganBooks, 2002.

Somers, Suzanne. *Ageless.* New York: Three Rivers Press, 2006.

————. *The Sexy Years: Discover the Hormone Connection: The Secret to Fabulous Sex, Great Health, and Vitality, for Women and Men.* New York: Three Rivers Press, 2004.

Bibliography

Female Sexual Dysfunction

Basson, R., et al. "Report of the International Consensus Development Conference on Female Sexual Dysfunction: Definitions and Classifications." *Journal of Urology* 163 (2000): 888–893.

Pauls, R. N., S. D. Kleeman, and M. M. Karram. "Female Sexual Dysfunction: Principles of Diagnosis and Therapy." *Obstetrical and Gynecological Survey* 60, no. 3 (March 2005): 196–205.

Dopamine and Libido

Bartlik, B. D., P. Kaplan, J. Kaminetsky, G. Roentsch, and J. Goldberg. "Medications with the Potential to Enhance Sexual Responsivity in Women." *Psychiatric Annals* 29, no. 1 (1999): 46–52.

Buffum, J. "Pharmacosexology: The Effects of Drugs on Sexual Function. A Review." *Journal of Psychoactive Drugs* 14 (1982): 5–44.

Hull, E. M., D. S. Lorrain, J. Du, L. Matuszewich, L. A. Lumley, S. K. Putnam, and J. Moses. "Hormone Neurotransmitter Interactions in the Control of Sexual Behavior." *Behavioural Brain Research* 105, no. 1 (November 1999): 105–116.

Pfaus, J. G., and B. J. Everitt. "The Psychopharmacology of Sexual Behavior." In F. E. Bloom and D. J. Kupfer (eds.), *Psychopharmacology: The Fourth Generation of Progress* (pp. 743–758). New York: Raven Press, 1995.

Rosen, R. C., and A. K. Ashton. "Prosexual Drugs: Empirical Status of the New Aphrodisics." *Archives of Sexual Behavior* 22 (1993): 521–543.

Shrivastava, R. K., S. Shrivastava, N. Overweg, and M. Schmitt. "Amantadine in the Treatment of Sexual Dysfunction Associated with Selective Serotonin Reuptake Inhibitors." *Journal of Clinical Psychopharmacology* 15, no. 1 (1995): 83–84.

Szczypka, M. S., Q. Y. Zhou, and R. D. Palmiter. "Dopamine-Stimulated Sexual Behavior Is Testosterone Dependent in Mice." *Behavioral Neuroscience* 112, no. 5 (October 1998): 1229–1235.

Taberner, P. V. *Aphrodisiacs: The Science and the Myth.* Philadelphia: University of Pennsylvania Press, 1985.

Dopamine and Fish Oil

Bourre, J. M, O. Dumont, and G. Durand. "Brain Phospholipids As Dietary Source of (n-3) Polyunsaturated Fatty Acids for Nervous Tissue in the Rat." *Journal of Neurochemistry* 60 (1993): 2018–2028.

Chalon, S., S. Delion-Vancassel, C. Belzung, et al. "Dietary Fish Oil Affects Monoaminergic Neurotransmission and Behavior in Rats." *Journal of Nutrition* 128 (1998): 2512–2519.

Chalon, S., S. Vancassel, L. Zimmer, et al. "Polyunsaturated Fatty Acids and Cerebral Function: Focus on Monoaminergic Neurotransmission." *Lipids* 36 (2001): 937–944.

Davidson, B. C. "Eicosanoid Precursor Polyenoic Fatty Acids Modulate Synaptic Levels of Dopamine in Ex-Vivo Slices of Rat Brain Striatum." *In Vivo* 17, no. 1 (2003): 83–88.

Delion, S., S. Chalon, D. Guilloteau, et al. "Alpha-Linolenic Acid Dietary Deficiency Alters Age-Related Changes of Dopaminergic and Serotonergic Neurotransmission in the Rat Frontal Cortex." *Journal of Neurochemistry* 66 (1996): 1582–1591.

Logan, A. "Neurobehavioral Aspects of Omega-3 Fatty Acids: Possible Mechanisms and Therapeutic Value in Major Depression." *Alternative Medicine Review* 8, no. 4 (2003): 410–425.

Zangen, A., R. Nakash, D. H. Overstreet, and G. Yadid. "Association Between Depressive Behavior and Absence of Serotonin-Dopamine Interaction in the Nucleus Accumbens." *Psychopharmacology* (Berl) 155 (2001): 434–439.

Zimmer, L., S. Delion-Vancassel, G. Durand, et al. "Modification of Dopamine Neurotransmission in the Nucleus Accumbens of Rats Deficient in n-3 Polyunsaturated Fatty Acids." *Journal of Lipid Research* 41 (2000): 32–40.

Zimmer, L., S. Delpal, D. Guilloteau, et al. "Chronic n-3 Polyunsaturated Fatty Acid Deficiency Alters Dopamine Vesicle Density in the Rat Frontal Cortex." *Neuroscience Letters* 284 (2000): 25–28.

Zimmer, L., S. Vancassel, S. Cantagrel, et al. "The Dopamine Mesocorticolimbic Pathway Is Affected by Deficiency in n-3 Polyunsaturated Fatty Acids." *American Journal of Clinical Nutrition* 75 (2002): 662–667.

Fish Oil and Nitric Oxide

Conner, William. "N-3 Fatty Acids from Fish and Fish Oil: Panacea or Nostrum?" *American Journal of Clinical Nutrition* 74 (2001): 415–416.

Goode, G. K., S. Garcia, and A. M. Heagerty. "Dietary Supplementation with Marine Fish Oil Improves in Vitro Small Artery Endothelial Function in Hypercholesterolemic Patients: A Double-Blind Placebo-Controlled Study." *Circulation* 96 (1997): 2802–2807.

López, D., et al. "Upregulation of Endothelial Nitric Oxide Synthase in Rat Aorta After Ingestion of Fish Oil-Rich Diet." *American Journal of Physiology. Heart and Circulatory Physiology* 287 (2004): H567–H572.

McVeigh, G. E., et al. "Dietary Fish Oil Augments Nitric Oxide Production or Release in Patients with Type 2 (Non-Insulin-Dependent) Diabetes Mellitus." *Diabetologia* 36, no. 1 (January 1993): 33–38.

Omura, M., et al. "Eicosapentaenoic Acid (EPA) Induces Ca(2+)-Independent Activation and Translocation of Endothelial Nitric Oxide Synthase and Endothelium-Dependent Vasorelaxation." *FEBS Letters* 487, no. 3 (January 2001): 361–366.

Fish Oil and General Health

Burgess, J. R., et al. "Long-Chain Polyunsaturated Fatty Acids in Children with Attention-Deficit Hyperactivity Disorder." *American Journal of Clinical Nutrition* 71, suppl. (January 2000): 327S– 330S.

Connor, W. E. "Importance of n-3 Fatty Acids in Health and Disease." *American Journal of Clinical Nutrition* 71, suppl. (January 2000): 171S–175S.

Conquer, J. A., et al. "Fatty Acid Analysis of Blood Plasma of Patients with Alzheimer's Disease, Other Types of Dementia, and Cognitive Impairment." *Lipids* 35 (December 2000): 1305–1312.

Heude, B., et al. "Cognitive Decline and Fatty Acid Composition of Erythrocyte Membranes—The EVA Study." *American Journal of Clinical Nutrition* 77 (April 2003): 803–808.

Hibbeln, J. R. "Seafood Consumption, the DHA Content of Mothers' Milk and Prevalence Rates of Postpartum Depression: A Cross-National, Ecological Analysis." *Journal of Affective Disorders* 69, no. 1–3 (May 2002): 15–29.

Hibbeln, J. R., and N. Salem. "Dietary Polyunsaturated Fatty Acids and Depression: When Cholesterol Does Not Satisfy." *American Journal of Clinical Nutrition* 62 (July 1995): 1–9.

Kris-Etherton, P. M., et al. "Fish Consumption, Fish Oil, Omega-3 Fatty Acids, and Cardiovascular Disease." *Circulation* 106 (November 2002): 2747–2757.

Laugharne, J. D. E., et al. "Fatty Acids and Schizophrenia." *Lipids* 31, suppl. (1996): S163–S165.

Morris, M. C., et al. "Consumption of Fish and n-3 Fatty Acids and Risk of Incident of Alzheimer's Disease." *Archives of Neurology* 60 (July 2003): 940–946.

Peet, M., and D. F. Horrobin. "A Dose-Ranging Study of the Effects of Ethyl-Eicosapentaenoate in Patients with Ongoing Depression Despite Apparently Adequate Treatment with Standard Drugs." *Archives of General Psychiatry* 59 (October 2002): 913–919.

Sears, B. *The Omega Rx Zone.* New York: ReganBooks, 2002.

Stoll, A. L., et al. "Omega 3 Fatty Acids in Bipolar Disorder." *Archives of General Psychiatry* 56 (May 1999): 407–12 and pp. 415–16 (commentary).

Chocolate

Di Tomasso, E., M. Beltramo, and D. Piomelli. "Brain Cannabinoids in Chocolate." *Nature* 382 (1996): 677–678.

Drewnowski, A., D. D. Krahn, M. A. Demitrack, K. Nairn, and B. A. Gosnell. "Naloxone, An Opiate Blocker, Reduces the Consumption of Sweet High-Fat

Foods in Obese and Lean Female Binge Eaters." *American Journal of Clinical Nutrition* 61 (1995): 1206–1212.

Melzig, M. F., I. Putscher, P. Henklein, and H. Haber. "In Vitro Pharmacological Activity of the Tetrahydroisoquinoline Salsolinol Present in Products from Theobroma Cacao L. Like Cocoa and Chocolate." *Journal of Ethnopharmacology* 73, no. 1–2 (November 2000): 153–159.

Birth Control and Female Sexual Function

Panzer, C., S. Wise, G. Fantini, D. Kang, R. Munarriz, A. Guay, and I. Goldstein. "Impact of Oral Contraceptives on Sex Hormone—Binding Globulin and Androgen Levels: A Retrospective Study in Women with Sexual Dysfunction." *Journal of Sexual Medicine* 3, no. 1 (January 2006): 104–13.

Warnock, J. K., A. Clayton, H. Croft, R. Segraves, and F. C. Biggs. "Comparision of Androgens in Women with Hypoactive Sexual Desire Disorder: Those on Combined Oral Contraceptives (COCs) vs. Those Not on COCs." *Journal of Sexual Medicine* 3, no. 5 (September 2006): 878-82.

Caffeine

Haleem, D. J., A. Yasmeen, M. A. Haleem, and A. Zafar A. "24h Withdrawal Following Repeated Administration of Caffeine Attenuates Brain Serotonin but Not Tryptophan in Rat Brain: Implications for Caffeine-Induced Depression." *Life Sciences* 57, no. 19 (1995): PL285–PL292.

Walton, C., J. M. Kalmar, and E. Cafarelli. "Effect of Caffeine on Self-Sustained Firing in Human Motor Units." *Journal of Physiology* 545.2 (2002): 671–679.

Testosterone and Female Sexual Function

Bachmann, G., et al. "Female Androgen Insufficiency: The Princeton Consensus Statement on Definition, Classification, and Assessment." *Fertility and Sterility* 77, no. 4 (April 2002): 660–665.

Berman, J., and L. Berman. *For Women Only.* New York: Henry Holt & Company, 2001, p. 112.

Guay, A., et al. "Serum Androgen Levels in Healthy Premenopausal Women with and Without Sexual Dysfunction: Part A Serum Androgen Levels in Women Aged 20–49 Years with No Complaints of Sexual Dysfunction." *International Journal of Impotence Research* 16 (2004): 112–29.

Panzer, C., S. Wise, G. Fantini, D. Kang, R. Munarriz, A. Guay, and I. Goldstein. "Impact of Oral Contraceptives on Sex Hormone-Binding Globulin and Androgen Levels: A Retrospective Study in Women with Sexual Dysfunction." *Journal of Sexual Medicine* 3, no. 1 (January 2006): 104–113.

Stark, K. D., and B. J. Holub. "Differential Eicosapentaenoic Acid Elevations and Altered Cardiovascular Disease Risk Factor Responses After Supplementation with Docosahexaenoic Acid in Postmenopausal Women Receiving and Not Receiving Hormone Replacement Therapy." *American Journal of Clinical Nutrition* 79, no. 4 (May 2006): 765–73.

Szczypka, M. S., Q. Y. Zhou, and R. D. Palmiter. "Dopamine-Stimulated Sexual Behavior Is Testosterone Dependent in Mice." *Behavioral Neuroscience* 112, no. 5 (October 1998): 1229–1235.

Serotonin and Exercise

Ernst, C., A. K. Olson, J. P. Pinel, R. W. Lam, and B. R. Christie. "Antidepressant Effects of Exercise: Evidence for an Adult-Neurogenesis Hypothesis?" *Journal of Psychiatry and Neuroscience* 31, no. 2 (March 2006): 84–92.

Serotonin and Libido

Clayton, A. H., et al. "Prevalence of Sexual Dysfunction Among Newer Antidepressants." *Journal of Clinical Psychiatry* 63 (2002): 357–366.

Montgomery, S. A., D. S. Baldwin, and A. Riley. "Antidepressant Medications: A Review of the Evidence for Drug-Induced Sexual Dysfunction." *Journal of Affective Disorders* 69 (2002): 119–140.

Stimmel, G. L., and M. A. Gutierrez. "Sexual Dysfunction and Psychotropic Medications." *CNS Spectrums* 11, no. 8, suppl. 9 (August 2006): 24–30.

Serotonin and Carbohydrates

Blum, I., Y. Vered, E. Graff, Y. Grosskopf, R. Don, A. Harsat, and O. Raz. "The Influence of Meal Composition on Plasma Serotonin and Norepinephrine Concentrations." *Metabolism* 41, no. 2 (February 1992): 137–140.

Lyons, P. M., and A. S. Truswell. "Serotonin Precursor Influenced by Type of Carbohydrate Meal in Healthy Adults." *American Journal of Clinical Nutrition* 47, no. 3 (March 1988): 433–439.

Wurtman, R. J., and J. J. Wurtman. "Brain Serotonin, Carbohydrate-Craving, Obesity and Depression." *Obesity Research* 3, suppl. 4 (November 1995): 477S–480S.

Vitamins and Minerals

Ali, H., M. Baig, M. F. Rana, M. Ali, R. Qasim, and A. K. Khem. "Relationship of Serum and Seminal Plasma Zinc Levels and Serum Testosterone in Oligospermic and Azoospermic Infertile Men." *Journal of the College of Physicians and Surgeons—Pakistan* 15, no. 11 (November 2005): 671–673.

"Iron Deficiency—United States, 1999–2000." *Morbidity and Mortality Weekly Report* (CDC) 51, no. 40 (2002): 897–899.

Om, A. S., and K. W. Chung. "Dietary Zinc Deficiency Alters 5 Alpha-Reduction and Aromatization of Testosterone and Androgen and Estrogen Receptors in Rat Liver." *The Journal of Nutrition* 126, no. 4 (April 1996): 842–848.

Prasad, A. S., C. S. Mantzoros, F. W. Beck, J. W. Hess, and G. J. Brewer. "Zinc Status and Serum Testosterone Levels of Healthy Adults." *Nutrition* 12, no. 5 (May 1996): 344–348.

Zheng, D., R. N. Upton, G. L. Ludbrook, and A. Martinez. "Acute Cardiovascular Effects of Magnesium and Their Relationship to Systemic and Myocardial Magnesium Concentrations after Short Infusion in Awake Sheep." *The Journal of Pharmacology and Experimental Therapeutics* 297, no. 3 (June 2001): 1176–1183.

PC Muscle Strength

Arvonen, T., A. Fianu-Jonasson, and R. Tyni-Lenne. "Effectiveness of Two Conservative Modes of Physical Therapy in Women with Urinary Stress Incontinence." *Neurourology and Urodynamics* 20, no. 5 (2001): 591–599.

Jonasson, A., B. Larsson, and H. Pschera. "Testing and Training of the Pelvic Floor Muscles After Childbirth." *Acta Obstetricia et Gynecologica Scandinavica* 68, no. 4 (1989): 301–304.

Ladas, A. K., B. Whipple, and J. D. Perry. *The G Spot and Other Recent Discoveries about Human Sexuality.* New York: Holt, Rinehart and Winston, 1982.

Masse, René. "The First Controlled Experimental Study Supporting the Theory That Myotonia Precedes Vasocongestion; Women Assigned to Kegel Exercise

Group Had Significantly Higher Sexual Arousal (Vasocongestion) Than Controls." Paper presented at Society for Scientific Study of Sex, New York, November 1981; Perry, J. D., and B. Whipple. "If Your Sexual Response is Poor, the Cause Could Be Weak PC Muscles." *Forum,* January 1981.

Perry, J. D., and B. Whipple. "Pelvic Muscle Strength of Female Ejaculators: Evidence in Support of a New Theory of Orgasm." *The Journal of Sex Research* 17 (1981): 22–39.

Protein/Carb/Fat and Testosterone

Anderson, K. E., W. Rosner, M. S. Khan, M. I. New, S. Y. Pang, P. S. Wissel, and A. Kappas. "Diet-Hormone Interactions: Protein/Carbohydrate Ratio Alters Reciprocally the Plasma Levels of Testosterone and Cortisol and Their Respective Binding Globulins in Man." *Life Sciences* 40, no. 18 (May 1987): 1761–1768.

Belanger, A., A. Locong, C. Noel, et al. "Influence of Diet on Plasma Steroid and Sex Plasma Binding Globulin Levels in Adult Men." *Journal of Steroid Biochemistry* 32, no. 6 (1989): 829–833.

Hamalainen, E., H. Adlercreutz, P. Puska, et al. "Diet and Serum Sex Hormones in Healthy Men." *Journal of Steroid Biochemistry* 20, no. 1 (January 1984): 459–464.

Howie, B. J., and T. D. Shultz. "Dietary and Hormonal Vegetarian Seventh-Day Adventists and Nonvegetarian Men." *American Journal of Clinical Nutrition* 42 (July 1985): 127–134.

Key, T. J., L. Roe, M. Thorogood, J. W. Moore, G. M. Clark, and D. Y. Wang. "Testosterone, Sex Hormone-Binding Globulin, Calculated Free Testosterone, and Oestradiol in Male Vegans and Omnivores." *British Journal of Nutrition* 64, no. 1 (July 1990): 111–119.

Soy and Testosterone

Habito, R. C, J. Montalto, E. Leslie, and M. J. Ball. "Effects of Replacing Meat with Soyabean in the Diet on Sex Hormone Concentrations in Healthy Adult Males." *British Journal of Nutrition* 84, no. 4 (October 2000): 557–563.

Nagata, C., S. Inaba, N. Kawakami, T. Kakizoe, and H. Shimizu. "Inverse Association of Soy Product Intake with Serum Androgen and Estrogen Concentrations in Japanese Men." *Nutrition and Cancer* 36, no. 1 (2000): 14–18.

Index

Index